HANDBOOK OF CARDIAC EMERGENCIES

HANDBOOK OF CARDIAC EMERGENCIES

Edited by
Dr Ian McConachie, *Consultant in Anaesthesia & Intensive Care*
Dr David Hesketh Roberts, *Consultant Cardiologist*
Blackpool Victoria Hospital

CAMBRIDGE UNIVERSITY PRESS
Cambridge, New York, Melbourne, Madrid, Cape Town, Singapore,
São Paulo, Delhi, Dubai, Tokyo, Mexico City

Cambridge University Press
The Edinburgh Building, Cambridge CB2 8RU, UK

Published in the United States of America by Cambridge University Press, New York

www.cambridge.org
Information on this title: www.cambridge.org/9780521265218

© Greenwich Medical Media Ltd 2000

The right of Ian McConachie and David Hesketh Roberts to be identified
as editors of this work has been asserted by them in accordance
with the Copyright, Designs and Patents Act 1988.

First published 2000
Digitally reprinted by Cambridge University Press 2010

A catalogue record for this publication is available from the British Library

ISBN 978-0-521-26521-8 Paperback

Cambridge University Press has no responsibility for the persistence or
accuracy of URLs for external or third-party internet websites referred to in
this publication, and does not guarantee that any content on such websites is,
or will remain, accurate or appropriate. Information regarding prices, travel
timetables, and other factual information given in this work is correct at
the time of first printing but Cambridge University Press does not guarantee
the accuracy of such information thereafter.

CONTENTS

PREFACE

This text:

- Is aimed primarily at trainees working in acute medical specialities. Hopefully it will also appeal to trainees in other disciplines who are involved in the care of patients suffering from cardiac emergencies. The text may also be of interest to coronary care and other nurses looking for information on modern therapy of cardiac emergencies. A basic knowledge of physiology and pharmacology is assumed as well as either a medical background or advanced nursing experience.

- May also be a useful 'aide memoir' for MRCP and other postgraduate examinations.

- Diagnosis is discussed only where relevant to therapy. Emphasis is on therapy based on modern physiologic principles.

- Is written by authors who are all experienced practitioners from a regional cardiac centre. The aim is to provide practical information on the management of common and/or important cardiac emergencies occurring in a district general hospital. The authors hope it will be useful at the bedside but emphasize that it, or any other book, is no substitute for experienced supervision, support and training.

- Some of the topics that are not emergencies in the strict definition of the term but are urgent cardiac conditions or problems in common practice.

- Does not aim to cover all cardiology practice and is not a substitute to the major cardiology reference textbooks.

- The format is designed to provide easy access to information presented in a concise manner. The authors have tried to eliminate all superfluous material. Selected important or controversial references are presented, as well as suggestions for further reading.

- The initial chapters introduce important concepts in pathophysiology and monitoring of the cardiac patient. Relevant cardiac pharmacology is presented in some detail. Later chapters cover the common or important cardiac emergencies as well as providing guidance on indications for referral to a specialist centre.

- Important information not readily available in similar texts, e.g. role and effects of mechanical ventilation, heart–lung interactions, the role of the right ventricle and cardiac manifestations of septic shock, are included.

- Many chapters are simply clinical reviews, others, e.g. catheter-based treatments for acute cardiac emergencies, represent 'state-of-the-art' reviews as of the end of 1999.

Ian McConachie and David Hesketh Roberts
Blackpool
February 2000

ACKNOWLEDGEMENT

Mrs Lynn Stanley, Department of Cardiology, supplied echocardiographs.

CONTRIBUTORS

Blackpool Victoria Hospital

Department of Anaesthesia & Intensive Care
Dr I. McConachie FRCA, Consultant
Dr C. Clarke FRCA, Consultant
Dr D. Kelly FRCA, Consultant
Dr M. Cardwell FRCA, Specialist Registrar
Dr M. Cutts FRCA MRCP, Specialist Registrar
Dr W. R. Macnab FRCA, Specialist Registrar
Dr D. Hume FRCA, Specialist Registrar

Department of Cardiology
Dr D. Hesketh Roberts MD FRCP, Consultant
Dr G. Goode MD MRCP, Consultant
Dr A. Chauhan MD MRCP, Consultant
Dr M. Brack MD FRCP, Consultant
Dr E. Lee MRCP, Specialist Registrar
Dr S. Bulugahapitiya MRCP, Research Registrar
Dr A. Brodison MRCP, Specialist Registrar
Dr R. Katira MRCP Staff Grade

Department of Cardiac Surgery
J. Au FRCP FRCS, Consultant

1

ACUTE CARDIAC
PATHOPHYSIOLOGY

CARDIAC CYCLE

The cardiac cycle describes the cycle of pressure and volume changes that result in sequential atrial and ventricular contraction. Events on both sides of the heart are similar. At resting heart rates systole (when ventricles contract) lasts for one-third of the cycle and diastole (when there is muscular relaxation and filling) for two-thirds.

The electrical activity of the heart initiates contraction of the atria and ventricles in sequence. The events described below apply to the left side of the heart.

- Mid-diastole – the AV valves are open. Atrial pressure is higher than ventricular pressure and blood flows from the atria into the ventricles.

- Late diastole atrial contraction occurs adding 20% to ventricular filling.

- Systole – ventricular contraction increases ventricular pressure. When this exceeds atrial pressure the AV valve shuts. This is known as isovolumetric contraction.

- Ejection – when ventricular pressure exceeds aortic pressure the aortic valve opens and blood is ejected.

- Late systole – ventricular muscle starts to relax and ventricular pressures fall below aortic pressure. Initially blood continues to be ejected because of the momentum imparted to it. At the end of systole blood flows back towards the ventricle causing the aortic valve to close. Blood is accommodated by the distension of the elastic aorta, which eventually recoils propelling blood towards the arteries. The volume of blood in the ventricle at the end of systole is the end-systolic volume.

- Early diastole – all the valves are closed. There is ventricular relaxation and falling ventricular pressure. This is known as isovolumetric relaxation. Eventually ventricular pressure is less than atrial pressure, the AV valve opens and blood flows from the atrium to the ventricle.

Similar changes occur on the right side of the heart. Pulmonary artery pressure is lower than aortic pressure, so right ventricular ejection precedes left ventricular ejection. Right ventricular ejection will go on for longer because the pulmonary circulation offers less resistance to blood flow than the systemic circulation and so the pulmonary valve closes after the aortic valve.

Clinical points:

- Loss of the contribution to ventricular filling by atrial contraction, e.g. in atrial fibrillation, can adversely affect cardiac function in failing hearts.

- The active force needed for ejection of blood from the ventricle is greater for a large ventricle than a small one. This is explained by the Law of Laplace, which states for a sphere $P = 2T/R$. Thus, ventricular cardiac muscle must generate a greater tension when the heart is dilated compared with a normal sized heart to produce the same intraventricular pressure.

- Tachycardia can cause ischaemia by reducing the time for ventricular filling and coronary blood flow.

- Cardiac output = stroke volume (litres) × heart rate (beats/min). Bradycardia can reduce CO and cause hypotension.

REGULATION OF STROKE VOLUME AND CARDIAC OUTPUT

Cardiac output (CO) is the volume of blood pumped by the ventricle/min:

$$\text{Cardiac output} = \text{stroke volume} \times \text{heart rate}$$

It ranges from 4 to 7 l/min in a normal adult at rest and can increase up to 17 l/min during exercise. CO is normally indexed to body surface area to allow comparisons of 'normal' CO between patients of different height and weight.

Stroke volume is the volume of blood ejected by the ventricle/heartbeat. It is the end-diastolic volume minus the end-systolic volume. Normally 70–80 ml for a 70 kg man at rest. Factors governing stroke volume include preload, afterload and the contractility of the cardiac muscle:

Preload

This is the volume of blood in the ventricle at the end of diastole, i.e. the end-diastolic volume. The Frank Starling Law of the heart describes the relationship between the end-diastolic volume and the resulting stroke volume. According to Starling, the greater the stretch of the ventricle in diastole the greater the resulting stroke volume. Thus, the heart has an intrinsic ability to control its own stroke volume by responding with a greater contractile force to the stimulus of increased diastolic stretch. This relationship is shown in figure 1

The degree of stretch of the myocardial muscle fibres when they begin to contract determines the number of actin–myosin cross bridges that can form that affects the degree of myocardial contraction achieved.

End-diastolic pressure is easier to measure than end-diastolic volume. For a compliant ventricle the two are related and end-diastolic pressure is used as a measure of preload. However, with reduced ventricular compliance (e.g. after a myocardial infarction) the pressure will be increased relative to the volume and end-diastolic pressure will overestimate preload. Preload gives information about the filling pressure of the heart. It does not give any information about blood volume.

Clinical points:[1]

- End-diastolic pressure in the RV is nearly equal to central venous pressure (CVP), which is the pressure within the right atrium and great veins of the thorax. It can be measured via a central venous catheter, using a manometer or transducer. Thus, the filling pressures of the right side of the heart can be determined.

- When resuscitating a hypotensive patient it should be ensured that they have an adequate proload, i.e. adequately filled with fluids before commencing inotropes or vasopressors.

- The CVP will not give any information on the filling pressures of the left side of the heart because the lungs are situated between the right and left sides of the heart. Pulmonary hypertension as a result of lung disease, mitral stenosis, left ventricular failure or increased pulmonary blood flow from right to left shunts will exacerbate the discrepancy. If either the RV or LV becomes selectively damaged, filling pressures on the two sides of the heart will differ. The pulmonary capillary wedge

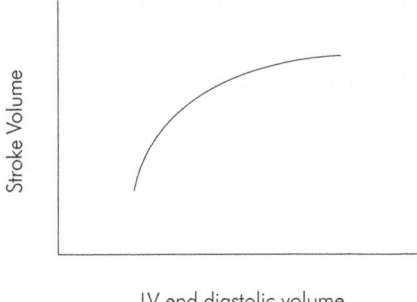

LV end diastolic volume

Figure 1 – Relationship between Lv end –diastolic volume and SV.

pressure (PCWP) is taken as a measure of end-diastolic pressure in the LV. This can only be measured with a pulmonary artery flotation catheter.

Afterload

This is the force that opposes ventricular muscle contraction, i.e. the ventricular wall tension that must develop to eject blood from the ventricle.

Afterload is increased by:

- Anatomical obstruction, e.g. aortic stenosis.

- Increased systemic vascular resistance (SVR).

- Decreased distensibility of the vascular system.

- Enlarged ventricle (Laplace).

- Increased blood viscosity, which is largely dependent on haematocrit. The greater the viscosity, the greater the resistance to flow.

- Decreased intrathoracic pressure (see Chapter 4).

Increased afterload will increase the workload of the heart and oxygen consumption and reduce stroke volume.

Afterload is reduced by:

- Reduced SVR.

- Vasodilator drugs.

- Anaemia.

- Increased intrathoracic pressure.

Clinical points:

- SVR accounts for about 95% of the resistance to ejection and is used clinically to estimate afterload.

- Blood pressure although convenient to measure is a poor reflection of afterload and gives no information about volume and flow to organs.

- Peripheral vasodilator drugs can improve the stroke volume of failing hearts by reducing afterload and ventricular work. Vasodilators also reduce preload via venous dilatation.

Contractility

This is the effective pumping ability of the heart muscle and is increased by:

- Increased sympathetic activity.

- Inotropes.

- Increased preload.

- Increased afterload – the Anrep effect.

- Increased heart rate – the Bowditch effect.

Contractility is reduced by:

- Decreased filling.

- Hypoxia and hypercapnia (although both will cause sympathetic stimulation).

- Acidosis and alkalosis.

- Electrolyte disturbances.

- Drugs, e.g. anti-arrhythmics.

Clinical points:

- The ejection fraction is often used as an indirect index of contractility:

  Ejection fraction = (end-diastolic volume – end-systolic volume)/ end-diastolic volume. The normal value is > 60%.

- Many drugs affect contractility and will be discussed throughout this book.

VENTRICULAR INTERDEPENDENCE (SEE ALSO CHAPTER 6)

Both ventricles share a common septum. Studies have shown that about 20–40% of the right systolic pressure and volume outflow result from left ventricular contraction.[1]

- If right ventricular end-diastolic volume increases, this shifts the septum towards the LV decreasing left ventricular diastolic compliance.

- Right ventricular volumes can increase with pulmonary hypertension.

MYOCARDIAL OXYGEN SUPPLY AND DEMAND

When myocardial oxygen demand exceeds supply myocardial ischaemia occurs.

The coronary circulation receives 5% of the CO. It has a high oxygen consumption and therefore a high oxygen extraction from the blood of about 70%.

Increased demand must be met by increased coronary blood flow. Hypoxia and adenosine are the most potent coronary artery vasodilators.

Factors affecting oxygen supply:

- Coronary blood flow which is dependent on:
- Coronary perfusion pressure (aortic end-diastolic pressure–left ventricular end-diastolic pressure).
- Length of diastole – at a heart rate of 70 beats/min diastole occupies two-thirds of the cardiac cycle. At maximum heart rates the cardiac cycle shortens, but diastolic filling is shortened to a greater extent than systole so that it only occupies one-half of the cycle. Perfusion of the coronary arteries occurs during diastole, a tachycardia will reduce the time for coronary perfusion and ischaemia can occur.
- Coronary vessel calibre – reduced by atherosclerosis. Chronic ischaemia allows some development of a collateral circulation. However, sudden occlusion of a vessel by thrombus results in cell death in the area supplied by that vessel unless protected by collateral circulation.
- Blood viscosity.
- Oxygen content of the blood which can be calculated using:

Oxygen content of blood = oxygen carried by Hb + oxygen dissolved in blood
$$= (\star 1.39 \times Hb \times saturation\%) + 0.0025 \times PaO_2,$$

where $\star 1.39$ is the Hufner constant. The volumes of oxygen carried by 1 g Hb. Figures vary according to whether it is measured *in vitro* or *in vivo*. The values 1.39 and 1.34 are the most commonly quoted ones respectively.

Factors affecting oxygen demand:

- Myocardial contractility and wall tension – contractile work accounts for the majority of myocardial oxygen consumption. There is a transmural gradient of wall tension that is greatest in the subendocardial region and least in the subpericardial region. Thus, energy requirements are greatest in the subendocardial region and may account for why the subendocardial region is more prone to ischaemia. Ischaemic myocardial metabolism results in the progressive loss of high-energy phosphates and progressive accumulation of catabolites. The transition from reversible to irreversible cell injury is likely to be influenced by metabolic rate.
- Heart rate.

ARRHYTHMIAS (SEE ALSO CHAPTER 2)

The electrical activity of the heart initiates contraction of the atria and ventricles in sequence. All cardiac myocytes have an inherent rhythmicity because of an unstable membrane potential. However, the sino-atrial (SA) node acts as the pacemaker of the heart as its intrinsic rate is faster than the rest of the heart.

The electrical impulse travels across the atria to the atrioventricular node (AV node) where transmission of the impulse is delayed, then rapidly down the bundle of His and Purkinje fibres to the ventricular muscle. Delay of transmission of the impulse at the AV node allows the ventricles to fill before they contract. Rapid impulse conduction down the Purkinje fibres allows simultaneous contraction of all the ventricular muscle fibres.

The principal mechanisms underlying arrhythmias are:[3]

- Conduction impairment – either slowed/blocked conduction, e.g. heart block or an abnormal pathway of conduction, e.g. Wolf–Parkinson–White syndrome.

- Re-entrant circuits.

- Enhanced automaticity – damaged myocytes develop an unstable membrane potential.

- Pathological after potentials – damaged myocardium may generate spontaneous after potentials after the action potential.

Cardiac arrhythmias are more common with:

- Hypoxia/hypercapnia.

- Electrolyte disturbances.

- Pre-existing cardiac disease.

- Certain drugs, e.g. inotropic drugs.

- Certain procedures, e.g. central line insertion where the catheter may directly irritate the heart muscle.

TISSUE OXYGENATION[4]

The function of the cardiorespiratory system is to deliver adequate oxygen to the tissues. Oxygen diffuses down a concentration gradient at the respiratory membrane and is then transported in the blood to the tissues. Most of the oxygen is bound to haemoglobin and a small amount is dissolved in the plasma.

Oxygen delivery (DO_2) is given by:

$$DO_2 = CO \times \text{arterial oxygen content (see above)}$$

Thus, oxygen delivery is dependent on adequate CO, haemoglobin concentration and saturation. Delivery of oxygen is controlled by the metabolic demand of the tissues.

Oxygen consumption is given by Fick's equation:

$$VO_2 = CO \times (CaO_2 - CvO_2),$$

where VO_2 is oxygen consumption, CO is cardiac output, CaO_2 is arterial oxygen content and CvO_2 is venous oxygen content.

Increases in demand are met by increases in blood flow and oxygen extraction. There is capillary recruitment thus increasing microvascular blood flow and increased extraction of oxygen from the blood thus reducing the mixed venous oxygen saturation (SvO_2). The saturation of mixed venous blood can be used to give information about tissue oxygenation although it needs to be interpreted with other clinical data. It can be measured continuously via an oximetric pulmonary artery flotation catheter or by blood sampling from an ordinary pulmonary artery flotation catheter.

If oxygen delivery becomes reduced, the metabolic demands of the tissues are initially maintained by increased extraction resulting in a reduced SvO_2. However, a critical point is reached at which anaerobic tissue respiration occurs and VO_2 falls. SvO_2 never falls to zero as there is an inability to extract all of the oxygen from the blood.

However, SvO_2 is a measure of global oxygenation and does not reflect oxygenation in individual organs. The normal range for SvO_2 is 68–77%.

Causes of decreased SvO_2 are:

- Low CO.
- Increased oxygen consumption, e.g. fever, exercise thyrotoxicosis.
- Decreased Hb.
- Low saturation.

Causes of increased SvO_2 are:

- Persistently wedged pulmonary artery flotation catheter (common cause).
- High CO sepsis, burns.
- Low VO_2, e.g. carbon monoxide methaemoglobin, sepsis, hypothermia cyanide toxicity.

Clinical points:

- If oxygen delivery decreases then oxygen extraction usually increases to compensate. However, in sepsis it appears that there is a decreased ability to extract oxygen.
- In patients with cardiac failure therapy may be titrated to SvO_2 as SvO_2 relates directly to CO.

PERIPHERAL CIRCULATION

The main determinants of blood flow are peripheral resistance and the pressure gradient. Given by Poiseuille's equation:

$$Q = \pi \times r^4/8 \times \eta \times l \times P_1 - P_2,$$

where Q is flow, $P_1 - P_2$ is pressure gradient, η is viscosity, l is vessel length, r is vessel radius and π is pi.

The distribution of blood flow is controlled by arteriolar tone as peripheral resistance is primarily dependent on the radius of the vessels.

Different tissues have different functions and this requires specialized vascular control. The kidney, brain and heart regulate their own tissue blood flow. Thus, blood flow remains constant usually between a mean arterial blood pressure of 60–140 mmHg. This is known as autoregulation.

Distribution of CO at rest:

- Liver 25%.
- Kidneys 22%.
- Brain 20%.
- Brain 14%.
- Heart 5%.
- Rest 14%.

This will alter under different circumstances, e.g. exercise and trauma.

Coronary circulation

Coronary oxygen extraction can increase to 90% in heavy exercise, but oxygen delivery mainly increased by increased blood flow.

Pulmonary circulation

Low vascular resistance so only small rises in pulmonary vascular pressure occur with increased pulmonary flow

Hypoxia in the lungs causes pulmonary vasoconstriction. If this occurs locally this improves ventilation perfusion matching in the lungs. However, global hypoxia will increase pulmonary vascular resistance that will reduce RV ejection and can eventually lead to RV failure.

Cerebral circulation

- Blood flow normally 50 ml/100 g/min.

- Blood flow is affected by:

- CO_2 – hypercapnia increases CBF; hypocapnia decreases CBF

- cerebral perfusion pressure CPP = MAP – CVP. Autoregulation occurs between a MAP = 60 and 140 mmHg but may be impaired with diseased and injured brains

- hypoxia – increased cerebral blood flow with a $PO_2 < 6.7$

- drugs, e.g. vasodilators

- hypothermia decreases cerebral blood flow

Renal circulation

Autoregulation occurs to maintain a constant renal blood flow. However, in haemorrhage this is overridden with vasoconstriction and redistribution of blood away from the cortex.

Skeletal muscle

Metabolic vasodilatation occurs during exercise. During strenuous exercise muscle blood flow accounts for up to 80–90% of CO and oxygen extraction increases from 25 to 30% at rest up to 80–90%. Extraction is facilitated by the presence of myoglobin in the fibres. During strenuous exercise anaerobic glycolysis predominates with the production of lactic acid. Post-exercise hyperaemia reverses the oxygen debt and washes out the accumulated lactic acid and other vasodilator substances.

PATHOPHYSIOLOGY

Hypertension

This increases afterload. If hypertension remains untreated the smooth muscle of the vessel wall hypertrophy, which causes narrowing of the lumen. The elevated resistance can then no longer be abolished by vasodilatation. Increased vascular resistance occurs resulting in end-organ damage. Hypertension results in increased myocardial workload and left ventricular hypertrophy. The increased end-diastolic pressure reduces coronary blood flow. The hypertrophied LV has an increased oxygen demand and angina and/or cardiac failure occurs.

Acute cardiac failure

When the heart is suddenly damaged (e.g. by a myocardial infarction) the contractility of the heart is immediately depressed resulting in reduced CO and increased systemic vascular resistance as a result of blood returning to the heart damming up in the veins. Intense sympathetic stimulation occurs almost immediately, which has an inotropic effect on the heart and causes vasoconstriction, thus increasing the mean systemic filling pressure and improving venous return to the heart. Increased end-diastolic volume caused by the reduced ejection fraction causes a compensatory increase in stroke volume by Starling's mechanism. Thus, the heart requires a greater filling pressure to maintain the same CO.

Chronic cardiac failure

Damaged myocardium as a result of myocardial infarction or haemodynamic overload, e.g. aortic stenosis results in left ventricular remodelling in an attempt to maintain CO and normalize wall tension.[5] This is achieved by activation of the renin–angiotensin system and hypertrophy of undamaged myocardium. These mechanisms may fail to normalize wall tension resulting in a further stimulus to remodelling and so a vicious cycle is set up. As the renin–angiotensin system is involved in this process, its inhibition by ACE inhibitors has been shown to decrease left ventricular volumes and to reduce mortality rate.

Stimulation of the renin–angiotensin system and altered renal haemodynamics results in fluid retention which increases mean systemic filling pressure and distends the veins reducing venous resistance so aiding return of blood to the heart. In severe failure there is excessive fluid retention that over distends the heart, reduces CO, and causes pulmonary oedema in left ventricular failure and peripheral oedema in right ventricular failure.

VALVE LESIONS

Aortic stenosis

Outflow obstruction to ejection causes LV hypertrophy and eventually LV failure. The LV requires high filling pressures and compliance is low thus left atrial and pulmonary artery pressures are high and RV failure occurs in end-stage disease. Coronary blood flow is reduced due to the increased left ventricular end-diastolic pressure and involvement of the coronary sinuses while left ventricular work increases. Ultimately LV contractility falls with left ventricular dilatation and reduced CO resulting in a low gradient across the valve in end-stage disease.

Management:

- Avoid hypovolaemia.

- Avoid tachycardia to allow time for ejection of blood from the ventricle.

- Avoid negative inotropes.

- Avoid peripheral vasodilatation as the CO is relatively fixed and the blood pressure may fall dramatically.

- Maintain sinus rhythm as atrial contraction is important to maintain adequate ventricular filling.

Aortic incompetence

Retrograde flow of blood through the aortic valve occurs during diastole causing LV dilatation and hypertrophy with a greatly increased stroke volume. Eventually compliance falls and left ventricular end-diastolic pressure increases with ventricular failure.

Management:

- Avoid hypovolaemia.

- Avoid bradycardia as regurgitation occurs during diastole.

- Avoid negative inotropes.

- Avoid increases in SVR as this will increase regurgitation.

Mitral stenosis

There is obstruction to ventricular filling resulting in left atrial hypertrophy and dilatation. Raised left atrial pressure results in increased pulmonary vascular pressures and reduced pulmonary compliance. The work of breathing is increased. If prolonged this results in pulmonary hypertension and right ventricular failure. In severe mitral stenosis the CO is fixed.

Management:

- Avoid hypovolaemia and vasodilatation, which reduce atrial and thus ventricular filling.

- Maintain sinus rhythm, as the contribution to ventricular filling by atrial contraction becomes important.

- Avoid tachycardia to allow time for ventricular filling.

- Avoid negative inotropes

Mitral incompetence

Mitral stenosis often coexists. There is retrograde flow of blood through the mitral valve resulting in left atrial dilatation. This results in left ventricular dilatation and hypertrophy and increased stroke volume. The distended and compliant left atrium accommodates large volumes with little change in pressure so pulmonary complications occur late in the disease.

Management:

- Avoid hypovolaemia.

- Avoid bradycardia, which increases regurgitation.

- Avoid negative inotropes.

ABBREVIATIONS, NORMAL VALUES AND EQUATIONS USED THROUGHOUT

- BSA = body surface area

- CO = cardiac output

- CI = cardiac index

- CVP = central venous pressure

- EF = ejection fraction

- EDV = end-diastolic volume

- ESV = end-systolic volume

- Hb = haemoglobin

- JVP = jugular venous pressure

- LAP = left atrial pressure

- LV = left ventricle

- LVEDP = left ventricular end-diastolic pressure

- LVF = left ventricular failure

- LVSWI = left ventricular stroke work index

- MAP = mean arterial pressure

- MI = myocardial infarction

- $PaCO_2$ = partial pressure of carbon dioxide in arterial blood

- PA = pulmonary artery

- PAFC = pulmonary artery flotation catheter

- PaO_2 = partial pressure of oxygen in arterial blood

- PAP = pulmonary artery pressure
- PCWP = pulmonary capillary wedge pressure
- PVR = pulmonary vascular resistance
- PEEP = positive end-expiratory pressure
- PVR = pulmonary vascular resistance
- RV = right ventricle
- RAP = right atrial pressure
- RVEDP = right ventricular end-diastolic pressure
- SA node = sino-atrial node
- SaO_2 = percentage oxygen saturation
- SvO_2 = mixed venous oxygen saturation
- SV = stroke volume
- SVR = systemic vascular resistance

Normal values

- CO = 4–6 l/min
- CI = 2.5–3.6 l/min/m²
- CVP = 0–8 cmH_2O
- EF = normally > 60%
- EDV = 75 ± 15 ml/m²
- ESV = 25 ± 8 ml/m²
- Hb = 13–17 g/dl (men); 12–16 g/dl (women)
- LVSWI = 40–80 g/m²
- PCWP = 6–15 mmHg
- PVR = 20–120 dyne s/cm²
- RAP = 1–7 mmHg
- SV = 80 ml
- Stroke work = 60–80 g
- SVR = 1000–1500 dyne s/cm²

Equations

CO = SV (litres) × heart rate (beats/min)

Cardiac index = CO corrected for body size = CO (l/min)/BSA (m²)

EF = left ventricular SV as a fraction of EDV = EDV – ESV/EDV

PVR = (mean PAP – LAP × 80)/CO

Stroke work = work done by the ventricle (usually left) = SV (ml) × (MAP – PCWP) × 0.0136

Stroke work index = stroke work/BSA

SVR = (MAP – CVP × 80/CO [80 is correction factor])

Further reading

Pinsky MR. *Applied Cardiovascular Physiology*. Berlin: Springer, 1997.

Priebe HJ, Skarvan K. *Cardiovascular Physiology*. London: BMJ Publ., 1995.

References

1. Lichtwarck-Aschoff M, Beale R, Pfeiffer UJ. Central venous pressure, pulmonary artery occlusion pressure, intrathoracic blood volume, and right ventricular end-diastolic volume as indicators of cardiac preload. *J Crit Care* 1996; 11: 180–8.

2. Santamore WP, Dell'Talia LJ. Ventricular interdependence: significant left ventricular contributions to right ventricular systolic function. *Prog Cardiovas Dis* 1998: 40; 289–308.

3. Boyden PA. Cellular electrophysiologic basis of cardiac arrhythmias. *Am J Cardiol* 1996; 78: 4–11.

4. Edwards JD. Practical application of oxygen transport principles. *Crit Care Med* 1990; 18: S45–8.

5. Blaufarb IS, Sonnenblick EH. The renin–angiotensin system in left ventricular remodelling. *Am J Cardiol* 1996; 77: 8C–16C.

2

ACUTE CARDIAC PHARMACOLOGY

SUPPORT FOR THE FAILING MYOCARDIUM

Strategies to support the failing myocardium and raise cardiac output include:

- Increasing myocardial contractility.

- Reducing afterload to reduce cardiac work.

- Increasing afterload to raise coronary blood flow thereby improving contractility.

- Increasing or decreasing preload to allow the myocardium to function in a more favourable part of the starling curve (see Chapter 1).

Many of these goals can be achieved pharmacologically. Inotropic agents increase contractile force of the myocardium at any given end diastolic volume. Vasoactive agents, diuretics, angiotensin-converting enzyme (ACE) inhibitors and opiates all achieve their effects by altering pre- or afterload. Each of these drug groups will be reviewed with reference to the important aspects of physiology relating to their action.

INOTROPES

Cardiac inotropes increase cardiac output and so improve oxygen delivery. This, however, is often at the expense of an increase in myocardial oxygen demand. They include endogenous sympathetic amines, which also vasoconstrict, and a range of synthetic compounds that aim to harness the beneficial effects of the endogenous amines without their vasoconstrictor effects. Improved contractility is brought about ultimately by an increase in myocardial intracellular calcium concentration, calcium being important for excitation–contraction coupling. Sympathomimetic inotropes do this by directly stimulating cardiac β_1-receptors that raise intracellular calcium via production of cyclic adenosine monophosphate (cAMP). Alternative strategies increase intracellular cAMP and/or calcium at an intracellular level.

Few direct sympathomimetic agents are pure inotropes. Most also have variable potencies at β_2, α_1, α_2 and dopamine receptors (table 1). This results in systemic vasoconstriction or vasodilatation and in variable effects on organ blood flow and other systems (table 2).

Inotropes are classified into inodilators or inoconstrictors.

Table 1 – Relative potencies of sympathomimetic agents.

Agent	α_1	β_1	β_2	Dopamine
Adrenaline	+++	+++	++	−
Dopamine	+++	++	+	+++
Noradrenaline	+++	++	−	−
Dobutamine	−	+++	+++	−
Dopexamine	−	+	+++	+
Isoprenaline	−	+++	+++	−

Table 2 – Adrenoreceptor effects.

Receptor	Effect
α_1	Cutaneous, muscle, splanchnic, coronary and renal vasoconstriction Glycogenolysis, lipolysis Intestinal relaxation Intestinal sphincter contraction Bladder contraction
α_2	Presynaptic inhibition of noradrenaline release from sympathetic nerves
β_1	Increased myocardial contractility Increased heart rate Increased conduction Increased myocardial excitability
β_2	Muscle, splanchnic, coronary and renal vasodilation Bronchodilation Glycogenolysis Intestinal and uterine relaxation
Dopamine	Splanchnic and renal vasodilation

INOCONSTRICTORS

Inoconstrictors are all endogenous catecholamines. As well as β_1 activity, they also have α_1-agonist activity resulting in peripheral, pulmonary, splanchnic and renal vasoconstriction. They are useful in low cardiac output states associated with vasodilatation perhaps secondary to a systemic inflammatory response to sepsis or following prolonged hypoperfusion.

Adrenaline (epinephrine)

Adrenaline is a very potent endogenous catecholamine. It is a potent α and β_1-agonist with moderate potency at β_2-receptors. β_1 effects result in an increase in heart rate, stroke volume, cardiac output and myocardial oxygen consumption. At low doses β_2 effects predominate with falls in systemic vascular resistance (SVR) and diastolic blood pressure due to dilation of muscle blood vessels. β_2-mediated coronary vasodilatation also occurs but may not be adequate to meet the needs of rises in myocardial oxygen consumption. As plasma concentrations rise α-mediated effects increase with renal, splanchnic, coronary and pulmonary vasoconstriction. Adrenaline's usefulness lies in low cardiac output states associated with vasodilatation, e.g. systemic inflammatory response syndrome, post-cardiopulmonary bypass and where less potent inotropes are failing to achieve adequate response.

Noradrenaline (norepinephrine)

Noradrenaline is a potent endogenous α_1-agonist with minimal α_2-receptor activity. It has moderate β_1 activity but almost no effects at β_2-receptors The result is systemic and pulmonary vasoconstriction resulting in a rise in both pre- and afterload. The effect on cardiac output is variable. Increase in afterload, by stimulation of the baroreceptor reflex, may result in a fall in heart rate and cardiac output. β_1 stimulation may maintain cardiac output in the face of this. However, better diastolic filling and/or better coronary perfusion (secondary to raised diastolic blood pressure) may result in a rise in cardiac output.

Noradrenaline is used predominantly as a vasoconstrictor, often to balance the vasodilatation produced by inodilators or where the need to increase the diastolic blood pressure outweighs the need to increase cardiac output.

Dopamine

Dopamine is the endogenous precursor of noradrenaline. Up to half its action is by biotransformation to noradrenaline, inhibition of noradrenaline re-uptake or noradrenaline displacement from nerve terminals. It is an agonist at dopamine$_1$, dopamine$_2$, α_1 and β_1-receptors, but lacks β_2 activity. Agonist activity is said to be dose-specific. At low dose rate (2–3 mcg/kg/min) the effects of stimulating dopaminergic receptors predominate resulting in increased renal blood flow, increased glomerular filtration rate, diuresis, natriuresis, splanchnic vasodilatation, reduced preload and reduced afterload. Heart rate and myocardial oxygen consumption is said to be unchanged. Medium dose rates (4–8 mcg/kg/min) see increasing β_1 stimulation, raising cardiac output. Further increases in dose rate stimulate α_1-receptors: SVR and PVR rise and any perceived benefit from dopamine receptor stimulation is lost as renal and splanchnic vasoconstriction ensues.

Low dose rate dopamine has often been used clinically in the belief that it may preferentially preserve renal blood flow and renal function in low cardiac output states. Despite this there is little randomized controlled trial data to support its use in this way. Dopamine may in fact cause a natriuresis from a direct effect on the renal tubules. Increases in renal blood flow may simply be the result of positive inotropic and chronotropic effects. A recent randomized controlled trial comparing low dose rate dopamine with low dose rate dobutamine in patients at risk of developing renal failure found a diuresis and natriuresis in the dopamine group.[1] However, creatinine clearance, perhaps a better indicator of renal function, remained unchanged in those receiving dopamine, whereas it rose in those receiving dobutamine. Its role in preserving renal function is therefore uncertain.[2]

INODILATORS

The inodilators are all synthetic agents, either catecholamine derivatives or phosphodiesterase inhibitors. While they posses varying direct or indirect β_1-agonist activity they lack the α_1 activity of the inoconstrictor group and have variable β_2-agonist activity resulting in vasodilatation. These agents are of value in low cardiac output states associated with vasoconstriction, achieving an increase in cardiac output both by an increase in myocardial contractility and by reduction in afterload.

Dobutamine

Dobutamine is a dopamine analogue consisting of a racemic mixture of stereoisomers with somewhat different receptor effects. Overall dobutamine is a potent β_1 and less potent β_2-agonist with only minimal α-receptor activity. It is a potent inotrope increasing stroke volume, cardiac output and, with increasing dose, heart rate. It produces systemic and pulmonary vasodilatation reducing afterload to both ventricles and increasing renal and splanchnic blood flow. Coronary vasodilatation results in improved myocardial blood flow and improved ventricular perfusion without increasing infarct size if used in acute myocardial infarction (MI). Dobutamine is said to be a more effective inotrope than dopamine in exacerbations of chronic congestive cardiac failure. This is because of its direct action compared with dopamine's part indirect action on sympathetic nerve terminals, which may become noradrenaline depleted in chronic myocardial failure.

Isoprenaline

Isoprenaline is a pure but non-selective β-agonist. It is a potent inotrope but its usefulness for this is limited by its propensity to cause marked tachycardia and tachyarrhythmias. Tachycardia and vasodilatation result in an increase in myocardial oxygen consumption and when used in acute MI increased infarct size may result. Isoprenaline is used most often as a chronotropic agent especially for temporary treatment of bradyarrhythmias and conduction defects.

Dopexamine

Dopexamine is actually a pure β_2-agonist with very little direct β_1 activity. It has no α activity but possesses some dopamine receptor action. Its inotropy results from inhibition of endogenous catecholamine re-uptake and from a baroreceptor-mediated reflex response to β_2-mediated vasodilatation that leads to an increase in heart rate. Because of this indirect route to increase in heart rate, dopexamine is less prone to precipitate tachyarrhythmias than the other catecholamines. Dopexamine reduces systemic and pulmonary vascular resistance and increases both renal and splanchnic blood flow. It may be used as an alternative to dobutamine and is used increasingly as a renal and splanchnic protective agent much as dopamine has been used in the past. Hypotension may limit its usefulness at higher doses.

Phosphodiesterase inhibitors

Phosphodiesterase inhibitors fall into three pharmacological groups: bipyridines (amrinone, milrinone), imidazole derivatives (enoximone) and benzimidazole derivatives (benzimidazole). They act by inhibition of the cAMP-specific phosphodiesterase III in vascular smooth and cardiac muscle. This enzyme is responsible for the breakdown of cAMP, levels of which rise, bringing about an increase in inotropy and smooth muscle relaxation. Some of the agents may also raise intracellular calcium by additional mechanisms. These agents raise stroke volume and cardiac output with little effect on heart rate. As a consequence they are less prone to cause tachyarrhythmias than the catecholamines. Systemic, pulmonary and coronary vascular resistances fall with increases in renal and splanchnic blood flow. Myocardial oxygen balance improves due to reduced afterload in the absence of a tachycardia. They have a longer half-life than the catecholamines. This means a loading dose must precede the infusion. Advantages of the phosphodiesterase inhibitors are that they may be effective where conventional inotropes fail especially in the presence of β_1-receptor down regulation. They also may encourage ventricular relaxation (lusitropic effect) if ventricular compliance is poor.

They have a role, particularly synergistically with direct acting β_1-agonists for acute ventricular support. However, they have been associated with increased mortality rate when used orally in the longer term.

Practical points in the use of inotropes and vasopressors

- Inotrope use is best guided by invasive haemodynamic monitoring. Bedside assessment of cardiac output and whether inodilation or inoconstriction is required is notoriously inaccurate.

- Most catecholamine inotropes are unstable in alkaline solutions.

- Inotrope stability is usually better in dextrose rather than saline solutions.

- Inoconstrictors cause skin necrosis if there is leakage from peripheral venous access. They are best given through a large central vein unless there are overriding clinical indications.

- Most catecholamines have a plasma half-life of 2–3 min. Steady-state is reached 10 min after changing an infusion rate. Changes in infusion rate are therefore best assessed for effect after 10 min. Plasma concentration is directly proportional to infusion rate.

- After prolonged stimulation of β_1-adrenoceptors, for example after several weeks of inotrope infusion in critically ill patients or in congestive cardiac failure where sympathetic tone is raised, β_1-adrenoceptors may become down-regulated so that reduced response occurs (tachyphylaxis). In this situation β_2-adrenoceptors become more important for increasing myocardial contractility.

VASODILATORS

Vasodilatation can be achieved through several mechanisms:

- Nitrovasodilatation – organic nitrates, sodium nitroprusside.
- α_1-receptor antagonism – phentolamine, prazocin, phenoxybenzamine.
- Direct action on vascular smooth muscle – hydralazine.
- Calcium channel antagonism – nifedipine, nimodipine, amlodipine.
- Angiotensin-converting enzyme inhibition – captopril, enalapril, lizinopril.
- Angiotensin-converting enzyme antagonism – losartan, valsartan.
- Opioid induced through central and indirect mechanisms.
- Potassium channel activation – nicorandil.

Nitrovasodilatrors

Both sodium nitroprusside and glyceryl trinitrate react with sulphydryl groups (e.g. glutathione) of proteins producing nitric oxide, an endogenous mediator that produces vasodilatation. They differ in the susceptibility of the arterial and venous circulations to their dilator effects.

Sodium nitroprusside

Sodium nitroprusside produces a balanced dilatation of arterial, venous and pulmonary vessels reducing both pre- and afterload. Given IV it has a rapid onset and offset of action (1–2 min) making it easily titratable and predictable. It may be useful in low cardiac output states associated with high filling pressures and vasoconstriction as is often seen in acute MI. However, the potential for reflex tachycardia and hypotension risks worsening of infarct size. It is also useful in acute hypertensive emergencies. Care is needed. Cyanide and thiocyanate metabolites may accumulate to cause toxicity with prolonged or excessive infusion rates.

Glyceryl trinitrate

In contrast to nitroprusside, glyceryl trinitrate has dose-dependent effects on venous and arterial circulations. At lower infusion rates it acts mainly as a capacitance vessel venodilator reducing venous return, preload and ventricular volumes. Higher infusion rates also produce increasing arterial dilatation reducing systemic and pulmonary vascular resistance. Half-life of 2–3 min allows rapid onset and titration of dose to blood pressure. Because of its effect on preload at lower doses it is especially useful in cardiac failure associated with pulmonary oedema, high filling pressures and dilated ventricles. It is also a potent coronary vasodilator so improving coronary perfusion. This combined with reduced ventricular volumes (reducing ventricular wall tension) has a beneficial effect on myocardial work versus oxygen availability. Glyceryl trinitrate is therefore also indicated for unstable angina and may reduce infarct size in acute MI. Prolonged use is limited by tachyphylaxis.

Nitric oxide

Nitric oxide can be administered directly by inhalation in ventilated patients. It then produces pulmonary vasodilatation, especially in ventilated areas of lung. This may, in certain situations, improve gas exchange by improving ventilation–perfusion matching. In the context of right heart failure secondary to pulmonary disease, it may be used to reduce RV afterload and improve cardiac output.

α-Antagonists

These agents are included for completeness, but their use in myocardial failure is limited. They produce arterial and venodilatation reducing pre- and afterload.

Reflex tachycardia and tachyphylaxis limit their usefulness in acute heart failure, although they may be of use in hypertension especially if secondary to excess catecholamines.

Direct arteriolar dilators

Hydralazine acts directly on arteriolar smooth muscle, probably by affecting calcium flux. There is some evidence that it increases intracellular cGMP levels so in fact it may act by similar mechanisms to the nitrodilators. It reduces pulmonary and systemic vascular resistances but has little effect on the venous circulation or preload. Reflex baroreceptor-mediated tachycardia may result and it should be used only with caution in acute MI.

Calcium channel antagonists

Calcium channel antagonists block the slow inward calcium channel found in cardiac and vascular smooth muscle, reducing calcium entry during cell depolarization. As a result they reduce myocardial contractility, cardiac conduction, peripheral vascular and coronary vascular tone. Different agents in the group have varying levels of effect on these systems (table 3). Their use in cardiac failure is actually limited by either negative inotropic effects or their tendency to cause reflex tachycardia. Their main roles are in the management of angina, arrhythmias and hypertension.

Angiotensin-converting enzyme (ACE) inhibitors

ACE inhibitors (captopril, enalapril, lisinopril) represent the greatest advance in the pharmacological management of cardiac failure in recent years. As well as bringing about symptomatic improvement, they are the only agents that have been shown to prolong survival in patients with moderate-to-severe congestive cardiac failure. In the longer term they promote ventricular remodelling and improve ejection fraction even in those patients with few clinical signs of cardiac failure. In

Table 3 – Calcium channel antagonists.

Drug	Conduction block	Negative inotropism	Coronary and peripheral vasodilation	Uses
Nifedipine Nicardipine Amlodipine	–	–	+++	angina hypertension
Verapamil	+++	++	++	AF SVT
Diltiazem	++	+	++	angina hypertension

low cardiac output states renal blood flow is reduced and sympathetic tone is increased. Both of these act as a stimulus to renal renin secretion. Resulting angiotensin II and aldosterone secretion then brings about vasoconstriction, salt/water retention, increased pre- and afterload. The result is a vicious cycle of increased cardiac work with further falls in renal blood flow and further increases in sympathetic tone. ACE inhibitors offer the opportunity to break this cycle by reducing angiotensin II and aldosterone levels. This brings about systemic and pulmonary vasodilatation reducing ventricular filling pressures and volumes. Cardiac work falls yet stroke volume increases. Increased renal blood flow together with reduced angiotensin II and aldosterone promotes diuresis. Intravascular volume depletion, often present following aggressive diuretic use, may result in profound hypotension requiring IV fluids.

ACE inhibitors also have other putative benefits:

- Inhibition of bradykinin breakdown.
- Improved vasodilator response to atrial natriuretic peptide.
- Sensitization of adrenoceptors to noradrenaline.
- Reduced post-MI remodelling of the ventricles.
- Free radical scavenging resulting in cardioprotection and reduced tolerance to nitrates.
- ACE inhibitors also have an established role in the management of hypertension.

In acute LV failure their potential for severe hypotension means their use is best reserved until the immediate crisis is resolving. The most common side-effect is cough. Renal failure, especially in the presence of renal artery disease or dehydration, may occur. Proteinuria, skin reactions and altered taste sensation may also be seen. Reduced aldosterone secretion promotes potassium retention and other potassium-sparing diuretics should therefore be stopped as dangerous hyperkalaemia may result.

Losartan and valsartan are specific angiotensin II receptor antagonists that result in similar effects to ACE inhibitors. They do not inhibit bradykinin breakdown and do not cause cough. They are useful in hypertension but their use in heart failure remains uncertain (trials ongoing).

Opioids

Morphine and diamophine are used in acute heart failure for vasodilator effects. In fact they have no direct vasodilator or inotropic action. Venodilation and some arterial dilatation probably result from a central effect on μ opioid receptors leading to a reduction in sympathetic tone. An additional effect may result from vasodilatation caused by release of histamine following injection of the drug.

Diuretics

The mechanisms of action of the commonly used diuretics are shown in table 4. Loop diuretics are of the most value in acute cardiac failure. They not only bring about a diuresis from their effects on the loop of Henle, but also increase renal blood flow and cause venodilation. It is actually this venodilation that is responsible for the immediate reduction in preload seen when frusemide is given IV in acute pulmonary oedema. Continued use of loop diuretics is associated with hypokalaemia and then they may be usefully combined with the potassium-sparing diuretics.

Potassium channel activators

Nicorandil is a newer agent promoting membrane stabilization by activating potassium channels. It causes both arterial and venodilatation. However, it has no role in acute heart failure but is indicated for management of angina.

ANTI-ARRHYTHMIC THERAPY

Cardiac arrhythmias are irregular or abnormal heart rhythms including bradycardias (< 60/min) and tachycardias (> 100/min) in adults. Understanding anti-arrhythmic therapy requires some knowledge of the electrophysiology of myocardial cell depolarization and the electrical conducting pathways involved.

Table 4 – Mechanisms of diuretic action.

Diuretic class	Example	Mechanism of action	Side-effects
Loop	frusemide bumetanide ethacrynic acid	inhibit Na/K/Cl exchange pump on thick ascending limb of loop of Henle	hypokalaemia
Thiazide	metolozone bendrofluazide	inhibit distal tubular Na reabsorption	hyperuricaemia hyperlipidaemia hyperglycaemia hypokalaemia
Potassium sparing	amiloride triamterene spironolactone potassium canrenoate	Inhibit distal tubular Na/K exchange binds aldosterone receptors in distal tubule	GI upset hyperkalaemia GI upset hyperkalaemia
ACE inhibitors	captopril enalapril lisinopril	reduces aldosterone and vasopressin secretion	cough renal failure hyperkalaemia

Electrophysiology

Heart muscle contraction is orchestrated by a system of conducting pathways originating in the sino-atrial (SA) node high in the right atrium. Conduction passes to atrial internodal tracts, atrio-ventricular (AV) node, bundle of His, the Purkinje network and finally to the contractile muscle cells of the ventricles. All myocardial cells have a resting membrane potential (RMP) and an automatic rate of membrane depolarization – a rate that is higher, the higher the cell lies in the conducting pathway. The RMP results from a selective difference in resting cell membrane permeability to sodium and potassium and to the different intra- and extracellular concentrations of these two ions. Resting permeability to potassium is relatively higher than to sodium. Potassium tends to diffuse out of the cell down its concentration gradient setting up a transmembrane potential that is negative with respect to the cell interior. The Na^+/K^+ ATPase transmembrane ion exchange pump maintains the high intracellular potassium and extracellular sodium concentrations needed to maintain the system.

Important differences exist between conducting and contractile cells. In the SA node the RMP is –60 mV whereas in the muscle cells it is closer to –80 mV. Cells lying in the conducting pathway have intermediate characteristics. The SA node automaticity results from instability of the Transmembrane Potential (TMP) (probably due to a gradual increase in sodium and calcium permeability and influx of these ions carrying positive charge into the cells). At a TMP of –40 mV, voltage-dependent slow calcium channels open and result in prolonged 100–200 ms depolarization. Repolarization results from the gradual closure of the calcium channels and the return of the TMP to that determined by the transmembrane potassium concentration gradient. In contrast the atrial and ventricular muscle have a resting TMP of –80 mV and depolarization is attributable to five phases:

- Phase 0 – rapid depolarization to +30 mV due to opening of voltage-dependent sodium channels and rapid sodium influx.

- Phase 1 – there is slight fall in the amplitude of the action potential resulting from the closure of the fast sodium channels and passive efflux of chloride ions.

- Phase 2 – prolonged depolarization, lasting 100–200 ms at +20 mV resulting from sustained opening of voltage sensitive calcium channels.

- Phase 3 – repolarization due to inactivation of the slow calcium channels and increased efflux of potassium. Cells are refractory to further stimulation.

- Phase 4 – resting transmembrane concentration gradients are restored by the continued activity of Na^+/K^+ ATPase.

Pharmacological strategies for the treatment of arrhythmias aim to address the causes by altering the transmembrane ion conductances with slowing of conduction, reduction in automaticity or increase in the refractory period.

ANTI-ARRHYTHMIC CLASSIFICATION

Singh and Vaughan Williams classified anti-arrhythmics originally into four groups (table 5).

Class I

Class I drugs block fast sodium channels reducing the maximum depolarization rate. This slows conduction and may increase refractory period. They have been subclassified by their effect on the length of repolarization (1a lengthens, 1b shortens, 1c has neutral effect on the duration of the action potential). Their effects are augmented by high extracellular potassium and reduced by a low concentration of the same. Indications vary with the agent but include both atrial and ventricular tachyarrhythmias. None of the drugs in this group have been shown to reduce mortality rate but they may in fact increase mortality rate in certain clinical situations, e.g. structural heart disease. They are best reserved for treatment of symptomatic arrhythmias in patients without structural heart disease.

Table 5 – Singh–Vaughan Williams classification of anti-arrhythmics.

Class	Mechanism of action	Effect	Examples
Ia		prolong repolarization	disopyramide procainamide quinidine
Ib	block fast inward Na channels, depressing phase 0 and slowing conduction	shorten repolarization	lignocaine mexiletine
Ic		little effect on repolarization	flecainide
II	reduce sympathetic action	reduced spontaneous firing, slowed conduction, prolonged AV node refractory period	atenolol propranolol sotalol
III	block delayed K rectifier current	prolong action potential duration and refractoriness	amiodarone bretylium sotalol
IV	block slow inward calcium channels	Reduce conduction velocity and increase refractoriness especially in the AV node	diltiazem verapamil

Class II

Class II agents act by reducing sympathetic action and are typified by β-blockers. β-Blockers exert their effects both directly by reducing the pro-arrhythmic effects of catecholamines released by the sympathetic nervous system and indirectly by reducing cardiac ischaemia. Block of β-adrenoceptors raises the threshold for ventricular fibrillation in ischaemic myocardium, reduces the spontaneous firing rate of the SA node and ectopic pacemakers, prolongs intranodal conduction and AV node refractory period. There is only moderate effect on refractoriness and conduction in the atria, ventricles and His–Purkinje system and no effect on action potential duration (except sotalol). β-Blockers are negatively inotropic and negatively chronotropic, reducing cardiac work. Their antihypertensive effects are less straightforward and may also involve baroreceptor resetting, presynaptic inhibition of noradrenaline release and inhibition of the renin–angiotensin system. They reduce early and late mortality rate following MI and are also used to treat hypertension and angina. Some β-blockers posses intrinsic sympathomimetic activity, local anaesthetic action, β-receptor selectivity or α-receptor blocking action. Those with intrinsic sympathomimetic activity may confer less cardioprotection following acute MI but are less likely to precipitate myocardial failure in those with precarious ventricular function. β-Blockers with α-blocking, vasodilating properties are being used in the management of congestive cardiac failure.

Class III

Class III agents prolong the duration of the action potential and refractoriness. Their chief action is to block the rectifier potassium current although all have other actions (e.g. sotalol, class II; bretylium, class II; amiodarone, all four classes)

Class IV

These drugs produce a dose-dependent block of slow inward calcium channels especially affecting cells whose depolarization depends on this, particularly the SA and AV nodes. They have no effect on infranodal conduction but are negatively inotropic, verapamil more so than diltiazem. They are used in paroxysmal supraventricular tachycardias including re-enterant tachycardias, and to control the ventricular rate in atrial fibrillation and flutter. Verapamil especially may cause bradycardia and AV nodal block. If combined with β-blockers verapamil may cause cardiac arrest. Negative inotropism means they may precipitate cardiac failure in at risk patients.

Selected anti-arrhythmic agents

Sotalol

Sotalol is a class III anti-arrhythmic, blocking potassium efflux during repolarization. It also is a β-blocker and has some class I activity. It prolongs atrial and ventricular action potential and refractoriness, slows SA node rate and prolongs AV node conduction. It is negatively inotropic (although less so than other β-blockers) and may precipitate heart failure. It is valuable treatment for a wide range supraventricular and ventricular arrhythmias including chemical cardioversion or control of the ventricular rate in atrial flutter and fibrillation. It is also used in ventricular fibrillation and tachycardia. It may however precipitate torsades de pointes and should be avoided in hypokalaemia, AV node block and prolonged QTc.

Bretylium

Bretylium blocks sympathetic nerves by depleting nerve terminals of noradrenaline. It prolongs repolarization, especially in the ventricles and Purkinje system with little effect on the atria. After parenteral administration it initially raises heart rate and blood pressure as the nerve terminals are depleted of noradrenaline. After 1–2 h, heart rate and blood pressure fall. Bretylium is said not to aggravate heart failure. Its main uses are in recurrent ventricular fibrillation and tachycardia especially following acute MI.

Amiodarone[3]

Amiodarone has effects in all Vaughan Williams classes. It blocks fast sodium channels, slow calcium channels, and also blocks the conversion of thyroxine to tri-iodothyronine. It reduces the maximum rate of depolarization, prolongs action potential duration, prolongs refractoriness, prolongs QT interval, prolongs AV node conduction and slows SA node discharge rate. It also has sympatholytic properties. The result is slowing of heart rate, increased AV node refractoriness and PR interval. There is some reduction in contractility (sympatholytic effect) and a systemic and coronary vasodilatation. Amiodarone is highly lipid soluble and as a result has a very large volume of distribution and half-life (30 days). This means a large loading dose is needed followed by reducing dose over several weeks. Accumulation occurs in lung, liver, fat, skin and other tissues. This accounts for many of the side-effects of corneal microdeposits, skin photosensitivity, slate grey discoloration, myopathy, neuropathy, pulmonary toxicity, disturbed liver function and gastrointestinal upset. Thyroid function tests become disordered and clinical hypo- and hyperthyroidism may ensue. Amiodarone's role is in both ventricular and supraventricular arrhythmias. It controls ventricular tachycardia and recurrent fibrillation. It reduces ventricular response in atrial fibrillation and flutter. It may also chemically cardiovert atrial flutter and fibrillation to sinus rhythm. It then helps to maintain sinus rhythm.

Adenosine

Adenosine is an endogenous purine active at, at least two receptors: A_1 and A_2 that inhibit and activate adenyl cyclase respectively. Its cardiac effects result from action at A_1-receptors and consist of reduced SA node automaticity and slowed AV node conduction. It is the drug of choice to terminate supraventricular tachycardias including re-enterant arrhythmias. It does not terminate atrial fibrillation or flutter although its AV node blocking action can be used to reveal flutter waves where rhythm determination is difficult. It is given as rapid 3, 6 and 12 mg IV boluses, ideally via a central vein. Side-effects of chest discomfort, dyspnoea, flushing, headache and nausea are short-lived since adenosine's half-life is < 10 s.

Digoxin[4]

Digoxin has two main effects on the myocardium:

- A direct effect: inhibition of Na^+/K^+-dependent ATPase. The result is a rise in intracellular sodium. Increased membrane sodium/calcium exchange leads to increased intracellular calcium.

- An indirect effect – stimulation of vagal efferents.

The results of these two effects are:

- Reduced SA node rate and therefore heart rate.

- Dose related AV node conduction block.

- Increased contractility (related to raised intracellular calcium and independent of cAMP). The duration of this effect is unlikely to be sustained for > 2–3 days and digoxin is not usually used for this effect.

- Reduced refractory period of atrial and ventricular muscle resulting in increased atrial ventricular excitability.

The main use of digoxin is to produce a degree of AV node block so reducing the ventricular response to atrial fibrillation and flutter. Reduced atrial refractory period means it may actually increase the rate of the atrial arrhythmia. Digoxin has a large volume of distribution and long half-life. A large loading dose (about 1.5mg over 24hrs) and small maintenance dose (62.5–250 mcg) is therefore needed. Elimination is by renal excretion. A reduced dose is therefore needed in the elderly and others with reduced renal function. Digoxin has a narrow therapeutic window so that monitoring of serum levels is important. Toxicity, which may be precipitated by hypokalaemia, results in atrial and ventricular extrasystoles, ventricular tachycardia and severe AV conduction block.

Magnesium[5]

Magnesium is the fourth most common cation in the body and is second only to potassium in terms of intracellular cation concentration. Deficiency is common in medical populations especially in critically ill patients and those treated with loop diuretics. Deficiency states are associated with increased atrial and ventricular excitability and a tendency towards arrhythmias. Pharmacologically, irrespective of serum levels, magnesium behaves like a calcium antagonist. Magnesium:

- Prolongs PR interval.

- Prolongs SA conduction time.

- Increases SA node refractory period.

- Causes systemic and coronary vasodilatation.

Magnesium is first line treatment for torsades de points and is increasingly used in acute supraventricular tachycardias including atrial fibrillation that may chemically cardiovert to sinus rhythm. The membrane-stabilizing effects of magnesium lead to its use following acute MI. Several small studies suggested a benefit, in terms of reduced arrhythmias when used in this situation, but larger studies (e.g. ISIS–4, > 58 000 patients) have now compared IV magnesium with placebo in acute MI showing no benefit from magnesium and those receiving magnesium actually suffered a higher incidence of heart failure and cardiogenic shock.[6]

Anticholinergic agents

These drugs (atropine, glycopyrolate) antagonize the effects of acetylcholine in the parasympathetic nervous system. As a result they cause mydriasis, bronchodilation, and are antisialagogue. Both may be used clinically to treat bradyarrhythmias and conduction block. Atropine has a faster onset and causes a greater tachycardia than glycopyrrolate. However, atropine may sometimes be associated with a worsening of bradycardia when given in low doses or intramuscularly (due to a central effect of vagal nucleus stimulation).

UNSTABLE ANGINA/ACUTE MYOCARDIAL INFARCTION (SEE CHAPTER 12)

Nitrates, β-blockers, calcium channel blockers and potassium channel activators have been discussed previously and will not be considered further here.

Aspirin

Aspirin reduces mortality rate when given in low dose (62.5–300 mg) following acute MI. It is likely that its benefit results from a reduction in platelet adhesion and aggregation. This is thought to prevent extension of coronary artery thrombus and thus limit infarct size.

In platelets thromboxane synthetase produces thromboxane A_2, whereas in vascular endothelium prostacyclin is produced. Thromboxanes encourage platelet aggregation and vasoconstriction whereas prostacyclins oppose platelet aggregation and cause vasodilatation. The balance between the production of these two agents plays an important part in maintaining the integrity of circulating platelets and vascular endothelium. Low-dose aspirin irreversibly inhibits cyclo-oxygenase. However, whereas vascular endothelium can regenerate cyclo-oxygenase, platelets, being anuclear, cannot do so. The balance is therefore shifted towards vasodilatation and inhibition of platelet aggregation. These effects of low-dose aspirin persist for up to 10 days until new platelets with functioning cyclo-oxyge-nase have been produced. Other effects of aspirin are also due to its inhibition of prostaglandin production and include anti-inflammatory, antipyretic effects and promotion of gastric ulceration.

Fibrinolytic agents (streptokinase, APSAC, t-PA)[7]

Formation of fibrin clot by the clotting cascade is normally opposed by a fibri-nolytic system. This system is initiated by activators released from damaged endothelium and results in the formation of plasmin from its circulating precur-sor plasminogen. Plasmin is a proteolytic enzyme that breaks down fibrin-dissolv-ing blood clot and preventing excessive extension of thrombus in the vascular tree. Fibrinolytic drugs break up thrombi by activating plasminogen to form plasmin. Their value in acute MI to reduce infarct size and mortality rate is well established. Greatest benefit is seen if they are give early but there are still benefits if given within 12 h and even up to 24 h following onset of acute infarction. As with any therapy the risks of use must be weighed against the benefits. They are con-traindicated if there has been recent bleeding, injury or surgery. They are also con-traindicated in coagulopathy, recent cerebrovascular accident and peptic ulceration and should be used with caution following invasive procedures and prolonged external cardiac massage.

Streptokinase forms a complex with plasminogen, converting it to plasmin. It is antigenic and may produce hypotension and a range of allergic reactions that may be severe. Using a slow infusion rate can reduce these. APSAC is anisoylated plas-minogen streptokinase activator complex. It is activated by hydrolysis and may cause less systemic thrombolysis. t-PA (tissue plasminogen activator) has a higher affinity for plasmin bound to fibrin so less plasmin is found in the circulation.

Further reading

Barnard MJ, Linter PK. Acute Circulatory Support. *Br Med J* 1993; **307**: 35–41.

Cody RJ. Pharmacology of angiotensin-converting enzyme inhibitors as a guide to their use in congestive heart failure. *Am J Cardiol* 1990; **66**: 7D–11D.

Feldman AM. Classification of positive inotropic agents. *J Am Coll Cardiol* 1993; **22**: 1223–7.

Nattel S. Comparative mechanisms of action of anti-arrhythmic drugs. *Am J Cardiol* 1993; **72**: 13F–17F.

Rutherford JD. Pharmacologic management of angina and acute myocardial infarction. *Am J Cardiol* 1993; **72**: 16C–19C.

References

1. Duke GJ, Briedis JH, Weaver RA. Renal support in critically ill patients: low-dose dopamine or low-dose dobutamine? *Crit Care Med* 1994; **22**:1919–25.

2. Chertow GM, Sayegh MH, Allgren RL, Lazarus JM. Is the administration of dopamine associated with adverse or favorable outcomes in acute renal failure? *Am J Med* 1996; **101**: 49–5.

3. Kowey PR, Marinchak RA, Rials SJ, Filart RA. Intravenous amiodarone. *J Am Coll Cardiol* 1997; **29**: 1190–8.

4. Campbell RW. Whither digitalis? *Lancet* 1997; **349**:1854–5.

5. McLean RM. Magnesium and its therapeutic uses: a review. *Am J Med* 1994; **96**: 63–76.

6. Seelig MS, Elin RJ. Is there a place for magnesium in the treatment of acute myocardial infarction? *Am Heart J* 1996;**132**: 471–7.

7. Kessler CM. The pharmacology of aspirin, heparin, coumarin, and thrombolytic agents. Implications for therapeutic use in cardiopulmonary disease. *Chest* 1991; **99**: 97S–112S.

3

SHOCK

This chapter aims to give a brief overview of clinical and pathophysiological aspects of shock. Many of the points covered will be expanded upon in later chapters.

Shock is an imprecise term for an acute clinical syndrome of tissue dysfunction secondary to inadequate tissue oxygen delivery. It is commonly accompanied by hypotension, but not necessarily so, a requirement for hypotension forming no part of the definition. Modern attempts at a definition focus on dysoxia with evidence of end-organ hypoxia and to this end some authorities insist on an elevated serum lactate as an integral part of the shock syndrome. Although shock itself is imprecisely defined its various subsets have been rigorously defined (e.g. consensus conference on septic shock[1]) in an effort to compare interventions in multicentre trials.

CLASSIFICATION OF SHOCK

Shock can be divided into different haemodynamic patterns. The widely accepted classification is that of Weil and Shubin.

- Hypovolaemic – usually due to haemorrhage or trauma but significant gastrointestinal fluid or 'third space' losses must not be overlooked.
- Cardiogenic – most commonly due to acute ischaemia.
- Distributive – main cause is sepsis but others include pancreatitis and burns.

Other causes include:

- Obstructive (extracardiac):

    tamponade

    tension pneumothorax

    aortic dissection

- Anaphylactic shock.

- Spinal shock.

- Traumatic – includes effects of tissue injury.

Although useful, this classification does not relate well to clinical practice where a mixed picture is frequent, for example the cardiac patient who has an anaphylactoid reaction during thrombolysis or the multiple trauma patient with subsequent bacterial translocation.

PATHOPHYSIOLOGY

Following an initiating event there is inadequate or ineffective perfusion, which results in organ dysfunction. Blood flow to any organ is related to perfusion pressure and also to the vascular resistance of the efferent or supplying vessel. Hypoperfusion occurs when there is an imbalance of the two forces, e.g.:

- If perfusion pressure fails to overcome high vascular resistance in cardiogenic shock.

- If vascular resistance fails to counteract low perfusion pressures.

- If there is a discrepancy in the interregional blood flow distribution in sepsis.

At a cellular level there is a cascade of reactions:

- Decreased delivery of oxygen and other nutrients, resulting in reduced ATP production.

- Disruption of the maintenance and repair of cellular membranes, followed by cellular swelling.

- Eventually permanent cell damage occurs, even if normal perfusion is restored.

- Past this point reperfusion injury may further prejudice recovery.

OXYGEN TRANSPORT IN SHOCK

The importance of the overall cardiopulmonary unit is emphasized in Chapters 1 and 4. The concept of oxygen transport has already been introduced in Chapter 1.

Tissue oxygen consumption (VO_2) is independent of oxygen delivery (DO_2) as delivery falls until a 'critical DO_2' is reached at which point there is physiologic supply dependence of consumption upon delivery. This point is well demonstrated in both experimental animals and patients and occurs at a DO_2 = about 330 ml/min/m². Below the critical DO_2 the mixed venous oxygen saturation will fall rapidly with corresponding increases in lactate, i.e. **shock** (figure 1).

In certain types of distributive, notably septic, shock this model does not hold as there is a failure of tissue oxygen extraction. Thus, mixed venous oxygen saturation (SvO_2) may remain high even at low levels of CI and DO_2. There may be a phenomenon of pathological supply dependency in sepsis whereby VO_2 is dependent upon DO_2, even above the critical DO_2 (figure 2).

This concept remains controversial as pathological supply dependency may simply be a result of mathematical coupling in the calculation of the variables.

Oxygen transport is of great theoretical interest but also has important practical applications:

- Because of the DO_2/VO_2 relationship, SvO_2 is a useful index of cardiac performance in cardiogenic shock and an adequate SvO_2 (60%) can be

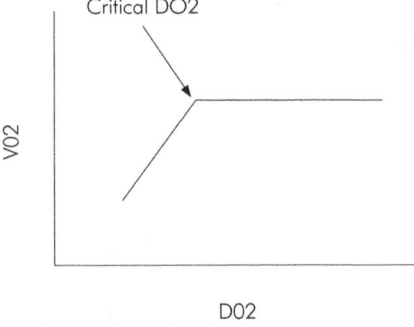

Figure 1 –Relationship between DO_2 and VO_2.

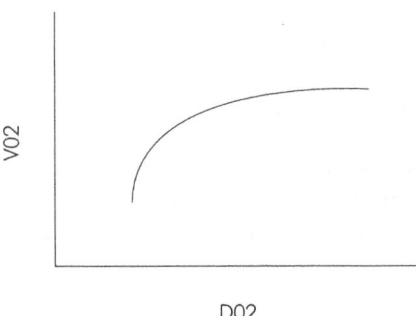

Figure 2 –Relationship between DO_2 and VO_2 and the pathological supply dependency.

used as a therapeutic end-point. In the setting of sepsis, however, continuous measurement of SvO_2 is not useful.

- Oxygen kinetics can be manipulated – if it is impossible to increase CI and DO_2 in a shocked patient then attempts can be made to decrease the oxygen demand and redistribute the available DO_2. This is part of the rationale for removing the work of breathing by mechanical ventilation in cardiogenic shock

CLINICAL PRESENTATION

Clinical presentation can vary because organs are affected differently not only between subjects, but also within the same individual. Presentation is dependent on factors such as the underlying cause, severity of the perfusion defect and premorbid organ dysfunction.

PHYSICAL SIGNS

- Hypotension – with a systolic blood pressure of < 90 or 60 mmHg below premorbid level.

- Tachycardia, thready pulse.

- Cool peripheries, clammy, pale and sweaty – due to sympathetic stimulation and vasoconstriction.

- Reduced conscious level – due to cerebral hypoperfusion.

- Oliguria – urine output < 0.5 ml/kg/h.

INVESTIGATIONS

- Haematology – full blood count, differential and clotting. The white cell count is often low in severe sepsis (and this is accepted in the definition). Cross-matching in haemorrhagic shock.

- Simple biochemistry – urea and electrolytes can help to assess both premorbid renal function and degree of end-organ involvement. Cardiac enzymes particularly troponin I levels are indicators of cardiac muscle damage.

- Arterial blood gases – to assess arterial oxygenation and also acid–base balance. The base deficit is a good marker of dysoxia and has been shown to track other allegedly more specific markers.

- Serum lactate – lactate rises due to inadequate perfusion and decreased liver clearance. Some authorities insist on lactic acidosis in their shock definition. Many hospital laboratories cannot easily measure lactate, but often the ICU analyser will have a lactate electrode. The lactate/pyruvate ratio may be a more sensitive marker of tissue hypoxia.

- Mixed venous saturation – can be measured from the pulmonary artery lumen (or displayed continuously using an oximetric technique). SvO_2 is useful in judging adequacy of CI and DO_2 if there is no oxygen extraction defect. In the critically ill SvO_2 must not be calculated using a standard blood gas machine. Shifts in the venous point of the oxygen–haemoglobin dissociation curve require it to be **measured** by co-oximetry.

- pH_i – gastric intramucosal pH (pH_i) is measured by a tonometric technique with a modified nasogastric tube. Low values (< 7.35) are an indication of inadequate splanchnic perfusion. pH_i has prognostic value and may act as a therapeutic goal in resuscitation.

Targeted investigations may range from microbiology, ECG, echocardiography, radiology and even a pregnancy test.

GENERAL PRINCIPLES OF MANAGEMENT

The aim of therapy is geared towards rapidly restoring tissue perfusion. Delay will allow hypoxic tissue damage and a downward spiral into multiple organ dysfunction (MODS). A basic ABC model of resuscitation should be employed.

Airway and Breathing (see also Chapter 4)

- Supplementary oxygen must always be administered using a high flow system.

- CPAP mask may be beneficial if pulmonary oedema is present.

- There should be a low threshold for intubation and intermittent positive pressure ventilation (IPPV). Obtunded patients aspirate – if in doubt protect the airway.

- IPPV reduces the work of breathing and also oxygen consumption.

Circulation

Assessment of cardiac function should be made:

- Heart rate and rhythm.

- Stroke volume (i.e. preload, contractility and afterload).

- Blood pressure

- End-organ perfusion (renal, cerebral and especially coronary)

- Aggressive circulatory resuscitation is mandatory if there is hypotension and signs of organ dysfunction.

The following steps are recommended:

Monitoring

- Non-invasive blood pressure (NIBP) monitoring is vital but has important limitations. NIBP readings may be spuriously elevated if the systemic vascular resistance is very low as the vibration in the arterial wall may 'rebound'. There should be a low threshold for arterial cannulation, which provides beat-to-beat blood pressure measurement and easy access for sampling. In the extremely shocked patient the femoral artery is often best (see Chapter 5).

- Urinary catheterization to assess renal dysfunction. The kidney has been described as the 'poor man's cardiac output computer'. Although the overall extraction of oxygen from the blood by the kidney is relatively low, the renal medulla (the metabolically active part of the kidney) extracts almost 80% of oxygen from its blood supply – the highest of any organ in the body. Thus, the kidney is especially at risk in shock of any aetiology.

- Central venous catheterization allows the measurement of right-sided filling pressures, which serve at least as an imprecise guide to volume status. Multilumen catheters facilitate the administration of vasoactive drugs (especially the emergency administration of noradrenaline to restore coronary perfusion while volume status is restored). A pulmonary artery catheter introducer is 8.5 French gauge and will allow rapid volume replacement and facilitate later pulmonary artery catheterization. Large bore multilumen catheters with integral introducer sheaths have recently become available.

- The relative merits of CVP and pulmonary artery catheter monitoring are described in Chapter 5. Currently there is concern that pulmonary artery catheterization or the treatment regimen consequent to catheterization might increase mortality rate, and utilization has fallen in the UK.

- Table 1 lists the basic haemodynamic patterns in the common causes of shock that may be used to guide therapy.

Table 1 – Common haemodynamic patterns in shock.

	CO	SVR	CVP	PCWP
Hypovolaemic	⇊	⇑	⇊	⇊
Cardiogenic	⇊	⇑	⇑	⇑
Septic	⇑/⇊	⇊	⇔	⇔

Therapy

- Large bore peripheral IV cannulation – short, large bore cannulae give best flows for volume loading.

- Fluid challenge – hypovolaemia must be treated promptly to restore organ perfusion and inotropes can have disastrous consequences in the presence of hypovolaemia. Thus, a fluid challenge is appropriate in nearly all circumstances unless obviously in gross pulmonary oedema. However, it should be carried out carefully with frequent assessment of response. Ideally patients should be volume-loaded along the Sarnoff curve – the relationship between pulmonary capillary wedge pressure (PCWP) and left ventricular stroke work index (LVSWI) – or the similar Starling curve as depicted in Chapter 1.

- Abnormal heart rate and rhythm may need to be corrected – including temporary pacing if required.

- Inotropic and vasopressor therapy may be required even as a temporizing measure. Patients with ischaemic heart disease must not be allowed to enter a downward spiral due to inadequate coronary perfusion pressure. Frequently vasopressors may be weaned or another vasoactive drug substituted as volume status improves.

- Specific treatments such as thrombolysis, antibiotics, chest drain insertion, surgery, etc.

Prognosis

Depends on the severity of shock, duration of tissue hypoperfusion, the underlying cause, degree of pre-existent organ dysfunction and likelihood of reversibility. Septic shock requiring vasoactive drugs carries a mortality rate of 40–60%,[3] and the mortality rate for cardiogenic shock post-MI remains 80–90%.[4] Prognosis may be improved if the duration of shock is kept to a minimum by early recognition and aggressive treatment. The concept of the 'golden hour' is well accepted with relation to trauma patients and is based on sound animal studies. A similar concept with its emphasis on prompt recognition and reversal of shock is undoubtedly applicable to other causes of shock.

Myocardial failure supervenes in all types of shock if the shock state persists. This myocardial failure is due a combination of acidosis, poor coronary perfusion and mediators released from ischaemic tissue including a myocardial depressant factor (MDF). Eventually there is progression to refractory shock with a loss of vasomotor tone, microcirculatory sludging, tissue hypoxia and cell death. As cellular and endothelial integrity fails, the situation may be compounded by 'translocation' of gut bacteria or endotoxin across the gut wall.

Further reading

Astiz ME, Rackow EC, Weil MH. Pathophysiology and treatment of circulatory shock. *Crit Care Clin* 1993; **9**: 183–203.

Jimenez EJ. Shock. In Civetta JM, Taylor RW, Kirby RR (eds) *Critical Care*. Lippincott-Raven, Philadephia 1997.

Edwards JD. Oxygen transport in cardiogenic and septic shock. *Crit Care Med* 1991; **19**: 658–63.

Shoemaker WC, Kram HB, Appel PL. Therapy of shock based on pathophysiology, monitoring, and outcome prediction. *Crit Care Med* 1990; **18**: S19–25.

References

1. American College of Chest Physicians/Society of Critical Care Medicine Consensus Conference. Definitions for sepsis and organ failure and guidelines for the use of innovative therapies in sepsis. *Crit Care Med* 1992; **20**: 864–74.

2. Rangel-Frausto M, Pittet D, Costigan M *et al*. The natural history of the systemic inflammatory response syndrome (SIRS): a prospective study. *J Am Med Assoc* 1995; **273**: 117–23.

3. Walters MI, Burn S, Houghton T *et al*. Cardiogenic shock: are HEROICS justified? *Circulation* 1997; **96**: 168A.

4

HEART–LUNG INTERACTIONS AND IPPV

In the past medicine encouraged a systems approach to disease. Thus, diseases of the heart would be taught in one unit and diseases of the lungs would be taught in another. Although not without merit, this approach has limitations. It is increasingly recognized that the organ systems work in series rather than in parallel, i.e. disease or therapy of one directly influences one or more other organs. Nowhere is this more apparent than with the heart and lung, which after all are connected by their vasculature and share the thoracic cavity. Indeed, the lung is the only organ that receives the whole cardiac output (CO). Forces acting on the lungs also act on the heart. Therefore, it is intuitively obvious that respiratory function and ventilation must have an effect on cardiac function. The team led by Pinsky has done much to investigate these issues and popularized the fact that the heart is a 'pressure chamber within a pressure chamber' (see further reading). This emphasizes that pressure applied to the lungs is automatically applied to and affects the heart. This has especial relevance to intermittent positive pressure ventilation (IPPV) and is discussed below.

This chapter attempts to give an overview of the ways in which the heart and lung influence each other with common clinical examples. The physiological effects of IPPV on the heart are explored again with clinical examples and implications. Some of the relevant issues are also explored in Chapter 6.

INTERLINKING OF THE HEART AND LUNGS

As stated, the heart is a pressure chamber within a pressure chamber. The most obvious effect of this is that as that as airway pressure increases, this pressure is transmitted to the right atrium and acts as a backpressure opposing venous return, i.e. venous return and CO decreases. During normal quiet respiration this effect is minimal but is measurable. The effects are of course magnified with IPPV when high pressures are applied to the lungs (see below). The other main effect of respiration on cardiac function is by changes in tidal volume. Again during quiet respiration these effects are minimal but with disease and IPPV effects can be clinically significant. Another phenomenon (of little clinical significance) is the decrease in vagal tone during inspiration producing the well-known phenomena of sinus arrhythmia.

CARDIOPULMONARY UNIT

If one takes the linkage of the heart and lungs to its logical conclusion and considers the overall cardiopulmonary unit, the main function of which is to deliver oxygen to the cells, then one must also take factors such as haemoglobin (Hb) and blood viscosity into account when assessing the patient. The increase in CO and minute volume with anaemia is a perfect example of the linkage of different organ systems to act as an overall cardiopulmonary unit. A recent report suggested that blood transfusion in patients with chronic obstructive pulmonary disease (COPD) reduced their work of breathing and improved their ability to wean off IPPV.[1] This is further support of the clinical importance of an overall cardiopulmonary unit. A different example in relation to COPD is given below.

It has also been noted that there are striking similarities between the way the heart and the lungs react to stress and in the way they fail! Table 1 illustrates the similarities.

CLINICAL EXAMPLES OF HEART–LUNG INTERACTIONS

Cor pulmonale

By definition, cor pulmonale means enlargement of the RV secondary to another disease process, usually of the lung or pulmonary circulation RV failure may be

Table 1 – Similarities between cardiac and respiratory failure.

Cardiac	Respiratory
Tachycardia	Tachypnoea
↓ Stroke volume	↓ Tidal volume
↑ End-diastolic volume	↑ FRC
Dyskinesia, hypokinesia and akinetic segments	Thoracoabdominal incordination
Pulsus alternans	Respiratory alternans
Heart block	Apnoeic attacks
Cardiac arrest	Respiratory arrest

Reproduced with permission from Scharf and Cassidy (1989), 739.

present and may be the sole cause of admission in many patients who are admitted to hospital with 'heart failure'.

Chronic obstructive pulmonary disease (COPD)

The association of COPD and right heart failure (cor pulmonale) has long been recognized. The COPD is usually advanced with severe airflow limitation (typical FEV_1 < 1 litre), chronic hypoxaemia and mild chronic pulmonary hypertension. These patients used to be referred to as 'blue bloaters' owing to the hypoxic-induced pulmonary vasoconstriction leading to pulmonary hypertension and RV failure. RV ejection fraction does not increase with exercise. Thus, both ventilatory impairment and RV dysfunction limit exercise tolerance.

The peripheral oedema found, even in the absence of true RV failure, may be partly due to airway obstruction and associated increased intrathoracic pressure impeding peripheral venous return. Frank RV failure may be precipitated in these patients by an acute infective exacerbation or ventilatory support and its development is an adverse prognostic sign.

Another cardiac problem in COPD patients relates to the common occurrence of arrhythmias, which have an adverse effect on prognosis.[2]

As hypoxaemia is such a key feature, it should perhaps not be surprising that long-term oxygen therapy (LTOT) is of major benefit. In fact, the British MRC trial of LTOT in the 1970s showed clear improvements in 5-year survival of COPD patients with pO_2 < 60 mmHg and prevention of progression of pulmonary hypertension.

The response to O_2 is variable:

- Some patients may acutely drop CO but overall oxygen delivery increases.

- Longer term, some may see a fall in Hb if polycythaemic, some may see a small decrease in pulmonary artery pressure and some patients increase RV ejection fraction and CO.

An interesting study found that survival was directly influenced by the degree of hypoxaemia. Non-survivors also trended towards a lower CO.[3] Other studies show lower venous pO_2 if oxygen delivery maintained by polycythaemia but with a relatively lower CO compared with relatively better maintained CO and lesser degrees of polycythaemia.

Thus, it is suggested that the development of polycythaemia may not be the best adaptive response and a failure to increase CO may influence survival. The implication is that therapies that maintain CO, e.g. vasodilators, may improve survival – but this has shown limited efficacy to date.

Massive pulmonary embolism (PE)

Acute circulatory failure is the commonest cause of death from PE. This is believed to follow acute RV failure secondary to the acute increase in RV afterload (acute cor pulmonale). Other factors include the development of RV ischaemia, decreased LV filling because of ventricular interdependence, hypoxaemia and vasoactive mediator release. Fluid therapy in acute PE is controversial. On the one hand, the further increase in right atrial pressure (RAP) should partially restore venous return and improve CO. However, further increases in RA and RV volumes may further impede LV filling. Inotropes may be useful by increasing ventricular contractility and vasopressors may improve right coronary perfusion. However, these interventions only serve to buy time for definitive intervention, e.g. thrombolytics or surgery.

Pulmonary hypertension

Pulmonary hypertension is usually chronic and, depending on the cause, progressive leading to chronic cor pulmonale and RV failure. Pulmonary pressure may be increased by occlusion, e.g. chronic, multiple pulmonary embolism, or due to vasoconstriction, e.g. pulmonary diseases. The prognosis of patients with pulmonary hypertension secondary to thrombo-emboli is directly related to the magnitude of rise in PA pressures, e.g. < 10% 5-year survival rate with PA pressures > 50 mmHg.[4] The prognosis for other causes of pulmonary hypertension is less certain and may even be worse for pulmonary hypertension secondary to COPD.

Status asthmaticus

Rarely acute, severe asthma is associated with haemodynamic compromise of a similar degree to that of cardiogenic shock.[5] The mechanism is thought to be one or more of:

- Dramatic elevations of intrathoracic pressure compromising venous return.

- Increases in LV afterload with the increased inspiratory efforts (see below on IPPV for a fuller explanation).

- 'Squeezing' of the heart by the hyperinflated lungs.

- Hyperinflation may also increase PVR.

Airway obstruction

A Mueller manoeuvre is a spontaneous inspiratory attempt against a closed airway. This leads to a decrease in intrathoracic pressure causing an increase in transmural pressure across the LV and increasing one reflection of LV afterload. (This is the opposite effect to the more commonly appreciated Valsalva manoeuvre.)

The clinical relevance of this is that airway obstruction occasionally is associated with the development of pulmonary oedema. Occasionally, following anaesthesia, laryngospasm has, again, resulted in pulmonary oedema.

Respiratory failure and the heart

Shallow breathing in respiratory failure can increase PVR, partly by collapsing alveoli causing a fall in diameter of extra-alveolar pulmonary blood vessels, and partly by development of hypoxic pulmonary vasoconstriction. The worsening PVR exacerbates the development of hypoxia and acidosis, which further worsens PVR! Thus, heart–lung interactions in respiratory failure can result in a progressive, downward spiral of the patient's condition.

Increased work of breathing and the heart

Any condition increasing work of breathing requires oxygen and energy. This requires increased blood flow and, in essence, the heart has to work harder. Thus, it is perhaps not surprising that respiratory failure causes a strain on cardiac function. The potential for myocardial ischaemia is also present especially when there is associated tachycardia and hypoxaemia.

Shock and respiratory failure

In severe shock, the reduced blood flow to the diaphragm coupled with the increased minute volume and respiratory energy expenditure causes respiratory failure – even in normal lungs. This is convincingly demonstrated in animal studies, e.g. much of the lactic acid accumulating in shock comes from the respiratory muscles.[6] IPPV, by reducing the work of breathing, lessens the blood lactate levels compared with spontaneous breathing. In cardiogenic shock the mode of death is often from respiratory arrest secondary to diaphragmatic fatigue, again due to the increased work of breathing.

Changes in CO and oxygenation

A pitfall is to wrongly ascribe a measured hypoxaemia to a respiratory illness when the true cause is cardiovascular in origin.

Falls in CO lead to a compensatory increase in oxygen extraction by the tissues. This results in a decrease in venous haemoglobin saturation (SvO_2). This directly results in a decrease in **arterial** saturation, especially in the absence of supplemental inspired oxygen. This, in itself, is one rationale for the administration of oxygen following myocardial infarction.

An exception to this effect is in the presence of physiological shunting through the lungs. Here a decrease in CO causes a decrease in the fraction of output shunting through the lungs and **no** change in pO_2.

Cough CPR

Although rare, there are reports of the patient's own cough maintaining sufficient CO to maintain consciousness following cardiac arrest. The pumping action may be due to the heart being 'squeezed' during each cough.

IPPV AND THE HEART

Cardiovascular effects

The two main effects of IPPV are:

- Lung volumes are increased – often significantly compared with spontaneous ventilation:

- Large TV causes a rise in pulmonary vascular resistance (PVR), which may lead to pulmonary hypertension and right ventricular compromise. This is due to the over-inflated alveoli causing compression of the alveolar blood vessels. The resultant increase in RV volume may impede LV filling (ventricular interdependence).

- In addition, large TV leading to hyperinflation releases factors into the circulation depressing the blood pressure. Animal studies suggest these to be prostaglandins.

- Hyperinflation can occasionally 'squeeze' the heart in the cardiac fossa causing falls in CO analogous with cardiac tamponade. This is occasionally seen in severe asthma or emphysema.

It has to be said that the exact clinical significance of these changes in most patients is open to doubt but high risk patients and those prone to hyperinflation, e.g. patients with emphysema may be more at risk.

- Intrathoracic pressure (ITP) is increased at all points in the respiratory cycle – compared with the 'negative' pressures generated during spontaneous ventilation:

- The heart operates as a 'pressure chamber within a pressure chamber' so it is therefore not surprising that changes in ITP affect cardiac function.

- Thus, changes in intrathoracic pressure are transmitted to the cardiac chambers during ventilation.

- Inspiration during IPPV increases ITP and therefore increases RAP relative to atmospheric pressure leading to a decreased gradient for venous return, reduced RV filling and reduced RV stroke volume. In addition, the increased ITP decreases the gradient across the LV that the LV has to work against – this is one definition of afterload. In other words decreased transmural pressure decreases left ventricular afterload. Both these effects tend to reduce intrathoracic blood volume. The increased RAP due to increased ITP may be misinterpreted as evidence of either fluid overload or cardiac failure if the mechanisms are not understood.

- Conversely, with decreased ITP as occurs with spontaneous breathing during inspiration the opposite is achieved, i.e. decreased RAP, increased gradient for venous return, increased RV stroke volume, increased LV transmural P and increased LV afterload. The combined effect is to increase intrathoracic blood volume.

- The decreased venous return and therefore decreased CO with IPPV is the major haemodynamic effect of ventilation in most patients. As it is related to ITP it is worse if the ventilator is set to provide either a high TV (high peak ITP) or a prolonged inspiratory time (high mean ITP). Positive end expiratory pressure (PEEP) also exacerbates the fall in venous return.

- Venous return and CO can be restored by either fluid infusion or sympathomimetic drugs both of which restore the gradient for venous return despite further increases in RAP.

Thus, increased ITP reduces not only reduces venous return (preload), but also afterload on the heart due to effects on transmural pressure. Which effect predominates depends on several factors, e.g. presence of hypovolaemia and, most importantly, the state of the heart. Any beneficial effect on afterload in the normal heart is limited by the fall in venous return. In the failing heart the CO is relatively insensitive to changes in preload (flat part of the Starling curve) but exquisitely sensitive to small reductions in afterload. Thus, in heart failure there may be beneficial effects on CO from increases in ITP with ventilation. In addition it will be crucial in the failing heart to avoid large falls in ITP as may occur during laboured spontaneous breathing as this can dramatically increase both preload and afterload producing pulmonary oedema.

With high ITP, right ventricular afterload usually increases due to increasing PVR and development of pulmonary hypertension. Thus, high thoracic pressures can reduce LV filling due to RV distension pushing the septum to the left to reduce LV chamber size (known as interventricular independence). This effect of excessive high thoracic pressure can counteract the beneficial effects on LV afterload.

Note:

- If pre- and afterload changes are controlled, IPPV, even with PEEP does **not** depress contractility and lower CO.[7]

- Despite attractive theoretical benefits, newer modes of IPPV, if delivering the same pressures and volumes, have exactly the same cardiac effects.[8]

- Cardiovascular consequences of IPPV are complex and vary in differing disease states.

Respiratory effects

- IPPV causes a potential increase in V/Q mismatch due to preferential ventilation of the non-dependant, poorly perfused lung regions. PEEP, in general, will improve oxygenation by recruitment of poorly ventilated lung regions.

- Decreased pulmonary perfusion if CO falls with IPPV causes an increase in alveolar dead space.

- Surfactant secretion is also reduced by prolonged IPPV.

Other effects

Humoral effects include an increase in ADH, renin–angiotensin and atrial natriuretic peptide lead to an overall retention of sodium and water. The oedema, particularly in the upper body, seen with prolonged IPPV is also promoted by inhibition of lymph and venous drainage from the upper body.

Beneficial effects

There is a considerable reduction in work of breathing and proportion of CO going to the lungs and diaphragm with a resultant increase in available CO and oxygen elsewhere. There are some that think this is the only definite beneficial effect of IPPV. Other beneficial effects include:

- Improvement in alveolar expansion particularly where there is lobar collapse often secondary to progressive hypoventilation and exhaustion.

- Oxygenation usually does increase but not necessarily in severe pulmonary disorders, e.g. ARDS.

- Suction or bronchoscopy easily remove secretions.

Harmful effects of IPPV

IPPV can damage the lung if:[9]

- excessive tidal volumes are employed ('volutrauma')

- excessive inspiratory pressures are employed ('barotrauma')

- in the absence of PEEP, repetitive opening and closing of alveoli cause damage by shearing forces ('low level barotrauma' or 'atelectrauma')

Inflammatory mediators may also be released which can cause a systemic inflammatory response (see also Chapter 7).

Monitoring considerations in the ventilated patient (see also Chapter 5)

When monitoring central venous or pulmonary capillary wedge pressures (PCWP) within the thorax, one must be aware that pressures transmitted to the vessels by the raised ITP during IPPV influence the accuracy of the measurements. Unfortunately it is too simple to assume that one can subtract the amount of the raised ITP from the measured vascular pressure to arrive at the true 'value'. Some authors in the past have even advocated taking the patient off the ventilator during measurement but this is not to be recommended.

To minimize the errors introduced by the raised ITP:

- It is the convention to measure PCWP at the end of expiration – when transmitted pressures are always at their lowest. For ventilated patients this is the lowest value displayed on the monitor screen when the pulmonary artery catheter is 'wedged'. For spontaneously breathing patients this is the highest value displayed on the screen (but still at end of expiration as ITP is lowest during inspiration as air is sucked in!) (figure 1).

- The catheter tip should be positioned in the lower third of the lung (higher up the alveolar pressure may exceed the pulmonary artery pressure during the respiratory cycle).

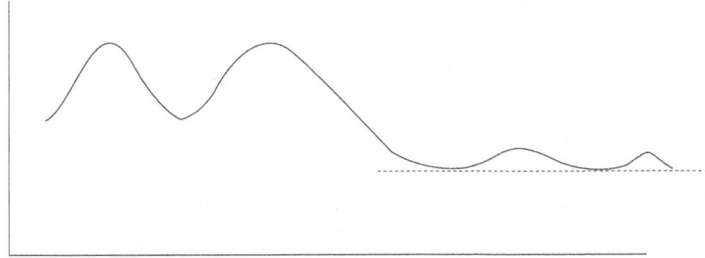

Figure 1 – PCWP during 'wedging' on IPPV. --------, End of expiration.

Cardiac output measurements

Cardiac output varies during the respiratory cycle due to the variations in venous return associated with the changes in ITP. These differences are magnified with IPPV. The question has been asked, 'should one measure CO at the same point in the ventilator cycle?' This begs the question, 'which is the correct CO; during inspiration or expiration? Of course they are both correct.

Practically, it is very difficult to synchronize CO measurements to the ventilator phases and, therefore, most practitioners aim to measure three or more outputs **randomly** through the cycle to get an average.

IPPV IN HEART FAILURE

As discussed above, the effects of IPPV on cardiac function are complex and differ according to the underlying state of the heart. However, there is additional evidence for significant, beneficial effects of ventilatory support in heart failure:

- Oxygenation is improved and hypercapnia controlled.

- Pulmonary oedema may be improved:

- alveolar fluid partially redistributed to the interstitial space further

- improving oxygenation

- prevention of oedema formation

- prevention of alveolar collapse in the dependant portion of the lung

  secondary to the 'weight' of the fluid filled lung

- Compressing or splinting the LV with regional wall motion abnormalities, the asynchronous region ejects more efficiently.

- In animal studies of cardiogenic shock, respiratory arrest is usually the mode of death due to diaphragmatic fatigue secondary to increased work of breathing. IPPV will eliminate the increased work of breathing.

- Face mask CPAP may be beneficial in cardiac failure and cardiogenic shock.[10]

- High-frequency jet ventilation synchronized with the cardiac cycle can increase intrathoracic pressure only during systole, reducing LV afterload while avoiding the reductions in preload during diastole. Early results with this technique show improvements in CO and oxygenation.[11]

However, although the above effects may be clinically significant, one must keep a sense of perspective. The effects may be relatively small compared with the percentage of the LV involved in cardiogenic shock.

CARDIAC PROBLEMS DURING WEANING FROM IPPV

The return to spontaneous ventilation may be analogous to a stress test! The beneficial effects of IPPV on cardiac function in patients with cardiac failure have been stated. Much of the clinical evidence for this is indirect, i.e. adverse effects of discontinuing IPPV on cardiac function. The evidence is:

- Patients with LVF and COPD may develop pulmonary oedema when IPPV is weaned with increases in PCWP.

- ECG recordings can reveal signs of ischaemia during weaning in many patients with coronary artery disease.

- A careful study of patients with COPD but no identifiable heart disease demonstrated reductions in LV ejection fraction in all patients during weaning which was not apparent in those patients on supported ventilation.[12]

The mechanisms proposed for these observations are:

- Increases in LV afterload with the decreases in ITP – especially if 'negative' intrathoracic pressures are generated during inspiration.

- Increases in intrathoracic blood volume as venous return increases with the decreases in ITP.

- Release of catecholamines during attempts at spontaneous breathing.

- Increases in the work of breathing, myocardial work and myocardial oxygen requirements.

- Increases in PVR with rapid, shallow breathing.

Thus, diuretics, nitrate infusions and/or ACE inhibitors may all be temporarily required during weaning. It also seems logical in these patients to 'support' the heart with inotropic drugs during weaning. In many patients the cardiac status is the main limiting factor for successful weaning. The variability of cardiac reserve and disease among patients may partly explain the poor predictive value of traditional tests of likelihood of successful weaning.

Further reading

Scharf SM, Cassidy SS. *Heart Lung Interactions in Health and Disease*. Lung Biology in Health and Disease, vol. 42. New York: Dekker, 1989.

Pinsky MR, The hemodynamic consequences of ventilation: an evolving story. *Int Care Med* 1997; **23**: 493–503.

Pinsky MR. Mechanical ventilation and the cardiovascular system. *Curr Opin Crit Care* 1996; **2**: 391–5.

References

1. Schonhofer B, Bohrer H, Kohler D. Blood transfusion facilitating difficult weaning from the ventilator. *Anaesthesia* 1998; **53**: 181–4.

2. Hudson LD, Kurt TL, Petty TL *et al*. Arrhythmias associated with acute respiratory failure in patients with chronic airway obstruction. *Chest* 1973; **63**: 661–6.

3. Kawakami Y, Kishi F, Yamamoto H, Miyatomo K. Relation of oxygen delivery, mixed venous oxygenation and pulmonary haemodynamics to prognosis in chronic obstructive pulmonary disease. *N Engl J Med* 1983; **308**: 1045–9.

4. Riedel M, Stanek V, Widimsky J, Prerovsky I. Long term follow up of patients with pulmonary thromboemboli: late prognosis and evolution of hemodynamic and respiratory data. *Chest* 1982; **81**: 151–8.

5. Raper R, Fisher M, Bihari. Profound, reversible, myocardial depression in acute asthma treated with high-dose catecholamines. *Crit Care Med* 1992; **20**: 710–12.

6. Aubier M, Vines N, Syllie G *et al*. Respiratory muscle contribution to lactic acidosis in low cardiac output. *Am Rev Resp Dis* 1982; **126**: 648–52.

7. Berglund JE, Halden E, Jakobson S, Landelius J. Echocardiographic analysis of cardiac function during high PEEP ventilation. *Int Care Med* 1994; **20**: 174–80.

8. Chan K, Abraham E. Effects of inverse ratio ventilation on cardiorespiratory parameters in severe respiratory failure. *Chest* 1992; **102**: 1556–61.

9. Slutsky AS. Lung injury caused by mechanical ventilation. *Chest* 1999; **116**: 9S–15S.

10. Bersten AD, Holt AW, Vedig AE *et al*. Treatment of severe cardiogenic pulmonary oedema with continuous positive airway pressure delivered by face mask. *N Engl J Med* 1991; **325**: 1825–30.

11. Pinsky MR, Marquez J, Martin D, Klain M. Ventricular assist by cardiac cycle-specific increases in intrathoracic pressure. *Chest* 1987; **91**: 709–15.

12. Richard CH, Teboul JL, Archambaud F *et al*. Left ventricular function during weaning of patients with chronic obstructive pulmonary disease. *Int Care Med* 1994; **20**: 181–6.

5

MONITORING

Monitoring may be described as the intermittent or continuous observation of a patient using clinical examination and appropriate equipment to assess progress of the condition. The most useful and reproducible monitor remains the thorough and repeated clinical examination by the doctor.

Not all critical care environments are the same, and all models of monitoring equipment are slightly different. The clinician must take time to become familiar with the equipment in his/her own hospital.

INVASIVE MONITORING

By definition a urinary catheter or a nasogastric tube is a form of invasive monitoring. However, by common convention, invasive monitoring is usually taken to refer to vascular cannulation. Mainly it is vascular pressures that are measured using pressure transducers although use of the pulmonary artery catheter permits many other measurements, calculations and sampling of blood. Before instituting invasive monitoring one must always ask: 'what are we monitoring and why?' The answer should be that something is monitored to do one or more of the following:

- Intervene therapeutically in emergency situations.
- Guide and plan future therapy.
- Establish diagnoses.
- Establish prognosis.

Monitoring is not a therapy in itself, which explains the argument that invasive monitoring does not in itself improve survival. Of course, any monitoring and measurements will not improve survival. Survival will only be improved if appropriate therapeutic measures are taken on the basis of the measurements taken. It should also be self-evident that the right measurements must be made and the information acted upon in the right manner. Much of the current debate about the usefulness of the pulmonary artery or Swan–Ganz catheter revolves around lack of knowledge on the part of the physician inserting the catheter and inappropriate therapeutic interventions based on the data obtained.[1,2]

Invasive monitoring has complications although careful technique and practice can reduce these. Therefore, one should always monitor non-invasively if possible. For example, the use of pulse oximetry has reduced (but not eliminated) the need for regular blood gas analysis, and automatic non-invasive BP measurement negates the need for direct arterial pressure measurements in many patients. However, in the critically ill patient, non-invasive monitoring may not suffice as discussed below.

In the discussion on direct arterial, central venous and pulmonary artery monitoring below, insertion techniques will not be discussed as they are best learnt at the bedside.

MONITORING MODALITIES

ECG

The standard 12-lead ECG is derived from the voltages measured from 10 electrodes attached to the patient: three 'limb' leads, six 'chest' or precordial leads and a grounding earth lead on the right leg. It is not always convenient to have all the chest leads attached to the patient. Indeed for monitoring it is rarely necessary.

An understanding of the anatomical area of the heart subtended by different leads permits rationalization of the 10 electrode set up:

- Of the precordial leads V_5, looking at the LV fed by the left anterior descending coronary artery, detects in the region of 90% of ischaemic changes in the ST segments (see ST analysis below).

- Leads II, III and aVF respond to ischaemia in the right coronary artery supplying the inferior aspect of the heart.

- As a consequence a five-lead set up of the four extremity leads and V_5 is commonly used as the standard continuous configuration. Viewing lead II and V_5 simultaneously allows inferior and anterolateral myocardial ischaemia to be detected.

- It is on occasions desirable to limit the monitoring hardware to a three-electrode system. During patient transfer and in isolated areas of the hospital the full range of leads may not be available. Under these circumstances the positioning of the three leads can be adjusted to optimize the view obtained.

Many configurations have been described including the positioning of leads on the patient's back to assist with atrial activity imaging. Two set ups are of particular use, these are the so-called CM_5 and CS_5 positions.

- CM_5 (central manubrium lead) – the right arm lead is placed on the manubrium. The left arm lead is placed at V_5, precordial position and the left leg lead is positioned in the normal way. This lead setting gives a close approximation of the V_5 lead when viewed on the monitor as bipolar lead I.

- CS_5 (central subclavicular lead) – the right arm lead is placed under the right clavicle. The other two leads are positioned as for CM_5. This setting allows bipolar lead I to read as 'V_5' as above but also allows bipolar lead II to be monitored on a second channel.

In the critical care setting the continuous ECG provides information on heart rate, rhythm, ST segment analysis and QRS complex configuration:

- Most acutely ill patients will present to hospital with a tachycardia (some may present with a bradycardia) and this in itself is reason enough for ECG monitoring. However, not all patients with a heart rate > 100 beats/min require continuous ECG monitoring. A static 12-lead ECG together with an appropriate history and examination will determine whether this is a 'normal' physiological sinus tachycardia that may not need continuous monitoring or a pathological rhythm producing an abnormal rate.

- Cardiac arrhythmias are common place across a wide spectrum of disease, and are by no means restricted to patients presenting with primary cardiac pathology.[1] Not surprisingly patients with primary cardiovascular problems will have the highest incidence of arrhythmia at about 90%. This falls to 44% in patients with acute trauma admitted to the general ICU. It is important that the critical care team is in a position to detect such arrhythmias promptly and act upon them to minimize the morbidity rate associated with undetected myocardial injury after trauma and as a response to other medical and surgical conditions.

- Specific evidence of myocardial ischaemia is available from monitoring the ST segments of the ECG. Clearly the goal of continuous ST segment analysis is the rapid diagnosis of myocardial ischaemia allowing its prompt treatment before irreversible myocardial damage occurs. Modern critical care monitoring systems usually incorporate ST segment analysis within the software. This system is applicable to coronary care patients, ventilated patients in the ICU and to patients on the operating table where swift response to developing ischaemia may save the patient progressing to a myocardial infarction.

- ST segment analysis is also of use as an indicator of the success or failure of thrombolytic therapy in the MI situation. Patients receiving thrombolysis following MI should have ST segment analysis for the first few hours after the event as failure of the ST segments to fall back to the iso-electric baseline may indicate failure of the thrombolytic agent to reperfuse the infarcted area and is associated with a poor prognosis as compared with the individuals in whom full ST regression occurs.[2]

Pulse oximetry

- It is often argued that in the last 25 years the single most important development in monitoring standards in the critical care environment has been the trend towards routine use of pulse oximetry.

- The pulse oximeter relies on the physics of spectrophotometry to allow the pulsatile flow of oxygen bound haemoglobin in arterial blood to be detected and differentiated from the surrounding tissue pigments and venous blood.

- Light of alternating wavelengths 660 and 940 nm is shone through the tissues and detected by a photocell that converts the absorption pattern to an electrical signal.

- The main unit processes the electrical signal generated from the probe. The information generated is converted to a digital saturation reading together with a plethysmograph waveform and an audible variable frequency pulse tone.

- The light emission/photocell detection unit is small and robust and comes in different designs for finger, ear or forehead use. (For a full explanation of the physics of oximetry, see the further reading).

- It is usual to measure peripheral arterial saturation by placing the probe on a finger. The toes may also be used. Under certain circumstances perfusion of the digits may not accurately reflect the central oxygen saturation in which case an ear probe attached to the lobe or a flat (reflecting as opposed to the conventional transmitting) probe placed across the forehead will be more useful.

- The detection of cyanosis is notoriously difficult particularly in anaemic, jaundiced, uraemic and dark-skinned patients. The pulse oximeter allows swift accurate and early detection of failure to oxygenate the blood.

- As stated above, the pulse oximeter detects the presence of oxygenated haemoglobin in the arterial system. Failure of oxygenated blood to reach the fingertip may occur anywhere along the path from the mouth and nose to the peripheral circulation. Falling pulse oximetry signals that a problem has occurred but it does not assist with localizing it.

As important as an indication of what can be learnt from the pulse oximeter is an understanding of what it does not monitor. The pulse oximeter is not a respiratory monitor. A patient with acute severe asthma and supplemental oxygen may have excellent saturation but a respiratory rate of 60 breaths/min and be on the verge of a respiratory arrest. The lesson from this example is of course that monitors do not replace the need for clinical examination.

Mixed venous oxygen saturation: SvO_2

This may be measured from a fibreoptic PAFC or by taking a sample from a PAFC and running it through a blood gas co-oximeter. The figure produced gives an indication of the global uptake of oxygen at tissue level. Interpretation of SvO_2 requires knowledge of cardiac output and oxygen delivery to the tissues. In general if the peripheral tissues are unable to utilize oxygen (e.g. sepsis, hypothermia), SvO_2 will rise. If the heart cannot deliver oxygen the tissues will extract as much as possible from what is available and SvO_2 will fall.

Direct arterial blood pressure measurement

The insertion of a small (common sizes are 20 or 22 gauge) Teflon-coated catheter into an artery, usually the radial, ulnar, brachial, dorsalis pedis or femoral are used, allows direct beat-to-beat assessment of the systemic blood pressure. Pressure transducers allow conversion of the mechanical pressure within the column of fluid attached directly to the blood vessel into an electrical signal that can then be displayed as a digital display and wave form. The presence of an arterial line also provides access for the measurement of arterial blood gas samples.

The pros and cons of this monitoring modality can be assessed by comparison with the non-invasive cuff pressure alternative.

Invasive arterial BP:

- Beat-to-beat control.
- Unaffected by rhythm.
- Automatic pulse measurement.
- Almost always possible.
- Accuracy unaffected by patient.
- Movement artefact clearly visible.
- Allows blood sampling.

- Susceptible to over and under damping.

- Requires training and practice.

- Potential ischaemic damage.

- Danger of accidental injection.

- Massive blood loss if disconnection.

Non-invasive BP:

- 'Stat' mode cycles about 20–30 s.

- Difficulty reading BP in AF.

- Not always available.

- Difficult in obese patients.

- Inaccurate in obese patients.

- Unable to read if moving.

- Blood sampling – not applicable.

- Over and under damping – not applicable.

- Easy to use.

- Cuff compression injury rare.

- Danger of accidental injection – not applicable.

- Blood loss if disconnected – not applicable.

- The decision to use invasive blood pressure monitoring is based on the clinical indication, together with an assessment of the ease with which it can be safely undertaken and the ability of the staff in the critical care area to look after the set up.

- It is probably inappropriate to run infusions of inotropic and vasoactive drugs without direct blood pressure measurement. It is also strongly advised that any ventilated patient have arterial access both for BP measurement and blood gas analysis.

- Common complications include local bleeding and infection. Serious complications include embolization and thrombosis and development of AV fistulae. Fortunately, serious complications are rare and can be minimized by choosing Teflon small-bore catheters inserted percutaneously.

- Intra-arterial pressure measurements are not always accurate, usually due to failure of calibration or wrong height of transducer. In general, the mean pressure is less prone to error, variation and excessive damping than the systolic and diastolic.

Central venous pressure monitoring

The central (or great) veins within the neck and mediastinum may be thought of as a manometer tube with four accessible branches – the right and left internal jugular veins and the right and left subclavian veins. The pressure measured within this 'venous manometer' is the filling pressure responsible for ventricular filling during diastole. The central venous pressure (CVP) may be judged clinically as the jugular venous pressure (JVP). This is very difficult to quantify and trends or sudden changes in the filling pressures are easier to assess directly.

Many critical care conditions cause the CVP to rise and fall. The usefulness of this monitoring system may be assessed from this list:

Conditions causing increase in CVP:

- Cardiac failure – if the RV cannot efficiently eject a stroke volume there will be increased back pressure in the systemic venous system.

- Cardiac tamponade – again if the RV is compressed by fluid in the pericardial sac back pressure in the great veins will cause the CVP to rise.

- Positive pressure ventilation – increased intrathoracic pressure produced during inspiration and the application of positive end expiratory pressure both result in elevation of the CVP.

- Fluid resuscitation – one of the commonest causes for CVP monitoring. To assess response to fluid resuscitation.

- Superior vena cava obstruction – owing to tumour or trauma to the root of the neck.

Conditions causing decrease in CVP:

- Hypovolaemia – any condition resulting in reduced venous return to the heart, e.g. exsanguination, sepsis, GI tract losses, sweating.

- Fall in intrathoracic pressure – at the end of a period of positive pressure ventilation and during spontaneous inspiration.

CVP monitoring should be considered in all critically ill patients in whom knowledge of the filling pressures of the right heart will assist in the resuscitation and maintenance of an adequate circulating volume to ensure optimal oxygen delivery.

CVP lines allow for the infusion of vasoactive drugs that would cause constriction of small peripheral veins. They may also be used for the infusion of irritant substances, e.g. parenteral nutrition and potassium.

After insertion of CVP lines via the above routes, a CXR must be obtained reasonably promptly both to rule out pneumothorax and also to check catheter tip position (SVC is ideal). If during and after CVP line insertion there is clinical deterioration of the patient the possibility of a pneumothorax **must** be entertained.

Long catheters can be threaded into the thorax via the basilic and cephalic veins in the antecubital fossae. The advantages are the little risk of bleeding and zero risk of pneumothorax. However, the complication rate is **higher** than that of other routes of central venous access. High infection rate and a high rate of thrombosis. The success rate is also low; 60% in some series.

Limitations of CVP monitoring or why one needs the pulmonary artery catheter

CVP reflects right atrial pressure, which is usually taken to reflect RV end-diastolic pressure. It does **not** necessarily reflect LV preload and also poorly correlates with blood volume. CVP is often used as a guide to LV function. Directional changes in CVP may reflect alterations in LV performance. However, if either ventricle becomes selectively depressed, or if there is severe pulmonary disease, changes in CVP will **not** reflect changes in LV function. Venous tone also influences CVP.

Pulmonary artery catheter

In 1970 Swan, Ganz and colleagues described a balloon-tipped catheter that could be inserted through the great veins via the heart to the pulmonary circulation. By means of the balloon the tip of the catheter could be isolated from the pressure generated by the RV.

Since its introduction into the critical care environment the pulmonary artery flotation catheter (PAFC) has attracted considerable 'adverse press'. This has ranged from concerns about the complications associated with the insertion and use of the catheter to the difficulties in interpretation and validation of the data obtained from it. More recently there has been a school of thought that implicates the use of the PAFC as deleterious to patient survival in the ICU environment.[3] These issues are touched on here and articles in the further reading.

The PAFC is 70 cm long and is inserted through a large bore IV introducer. The design of the catheter may vary between manufacturers but consistent features include:

- Gradations along the length in 10 cm.

- Ports at the proximal end:

- connection to the balloon allowing the use of a 2 ml syringe to inflate the balloon

- distal lumen port allowing connection to the pressure transducer system

- proximal lumen port – opens some distance from the tip

- Various additions and modifications including further infusion ports, CVP monitoring port, thermistor connection, heating coil, continuous venous oximetry cable and pacing facilities.

The information gained from the PAFC is of three types:

- Pressures derived from catheter placement.

- Measurement of cardiac output

- Mathematically derived data

PRESSURES DERIVED FROM CATHETER PLACEMENT

During the insertion of the PAFC the pressures produced from the transduced catheter tip as it 'floats' (balloon inflated during insertion) through the right heart are: CVP, right atrial pressure, right ventricular pressure, pulmonary artery pressure and pulmonary capillary wedge pressure (PCWP). PCWP is measured by the tip of the catheter when the forward pressure from the RV is obstructed by the balloon (this pressure should be measured for < 30 s at a time as the pulmonary blood flow is ceased down stream of the inflated balloon making pulmonary infarction a possibility). PCWP is also known as the pulmonary artery occlusion pressure (PAOP).

Provided the tip of the catheter is contained within a continuous column of blood between it and the LV, then at the end of diastole with the mitral valve open, the PAFC measures the left ventricular end-diastolic pressure (LVEDP). From Starling's law, the force of contraction of the LV is dependent on the degree of muscle fibre stretch during diastolic filling. Thus, provided the ventricle wall is of normal compliance the pressure developed within the ventricle at end-diastole is directly proportional to the ventricular volume (LVEDV) and hence to preload. Under these conditions, PCWP directly reflects LVEDV.

Clearly there are situations in which the above relationship does not hold.

- In patients undergoing positive pressure mechanical ventilation with high airway pressures the alveolar pressure may exceed pulmonary venule pressure. In this state the continuous column of blood is 'broken' and the wedged PAFC is measuring the alveolar pressure.

- Mitral valve disease affects PCWP. Mitral stenosis causes a large back pressure ('a' wave) on the PCWP trace as the atrium contracts against the stenotic valve. Mitral regurgitation causes a large 'v' wave as the ventricular outflow passes back up the pulmonary venous system.

- The compliance of the ventricle wall is altered in states of cardiac and systemic disease. Myocardial infarction, cardiac tamponade, aortic valve disease, the cardiomyopathies and systemic sepsis all cause the PCWP not to reflect LVEDV. This observation may be used clinically to assess the severity of the causative condition.

Cardiac output

If a known volume of a substance (tracer) is injected into the right atrium, the alteration in the concentration of the tracer as it passes the sensor in the PAFC over time, may be used to calculate cardiac output. The tracer used clinically is cold saline and the temperature washout curve is processed by the monitoring unit using the Stewart–Hamilton equation to integrate the area under the curve to produce the cardiac output. (Modern catheters can measure cardiac output continuously by the same principle but in reverse, i.e. heated filament to produce small increases in blood temperature).

Sources of error within this system are that the cold tracer is dissipated to nonblood structures, i.e.. the catheter and the vessel walls, producing exaggerated values. Cardiac output measurement varies during the respiratory cycle, being greatest at end expiration. This difference is exaggerated by the use of high inflation pressures during IPPV.

Mathematically derived data

From the measured data produced by the PAFC together with knowledge of the systemic mean blood pressure (from the arterial line) and the central venous pressure (from the CVP line) a further set of derived data may be produced:

- Systemic and pulmonary vascular resistance.

- LV and RV stroke work.

- LV and RV stroke volume.

- Right ventricular ejection fraction (rapid response thermistor catheters only).

Although mathematical formulae for each of the above figures exists (see Chapter 1), modern monitoring systems calculate them automatically.

There is without doubt a great deal of information that can be gained about the critically ill patient from a PAFC. Perhaps more so than with the other monitoring modalities it is vital that the limitations and potential errors within the data produced are fully understood so the decision to use a PAFC can be made appropriately.[4] If the PAFC is used simply to watch the unabated deterioration of a critically ill patient, then the decision to use it is questionable. However, if the catheter is inserted early in the course of critical disease it can provide the clinician with the information needed to help tailor fluid, vasoactive and inotropic therapy appropriately.

INDICATIONS

- Monitor preload.

- Optimize preload before the use of inotropes.

- Pulmonary oedema not responsive to simple measures or where therapy produces hypotension.

- Shock.

- Complicated MI.

- To enable manipulation of oxygen transport variables.

- Differentiate cardiogenic and non-cardiogenic pulmonary oedema.

- More rarely, after acute MI, to differentiate between acute VSD and mitral regurgitation.

- May be inserted prophylactically for high-risk surgery especially cardiac surgery

COMPLICATIONS

During insertion – same as for CVP depending on site chosen:

- Carotid haematoma

- Pneumothorax

- Haemothorax

- Neurological injury

- Haemorrhage

- Lymphatic injury

During passage of the catheter:

- Arrhythmias

- Intracardiac knotting

- Cardiac or PA perforation

Catheter *in situ*:

- Pulmonary embolism and infarction
- Valve damage
- Thrombocytopenia (not such a problem with modern catheters)
- Endocarditis
- PA rupture
- Inaccurate measurements and false interpretations

Hints on safe use of PAFC

- Balance risk versus benefit.
- Slowly inflate balloon while watching waveform.
- On wedging trace stop further inflation of balloon.
- If catheter overwedges, immediately deflate balloon and withdraw catheter 1–2 cm.
- Minimize duration of balloon inflation.
- If balloon inflates with < 1.5 ml air, withdraw 1 cm.
- Continuously monitor PA trace for spontaneous migration and wedging.
- Minimize number of wedgings in patients with pulmonary hypertension.

Further reading

Coalition for Critical Care Excellence: Consensus Conference on Physiologic Monitoring Devices. Standards of evidence for the safety and effectiveness of critical care monitoring devices and related interventions. *Crit Care Med* 1995; **23**: 1756–63.

Levy MM. Monitoring cardiac function and tissue perfusion. *Crit Care Clin* 1996; **12**: 771–1043.

Moyle J. *Pulse Oximetry*. London: BMJ Publ., 1994.

Shephard JN, Brecker SJ, Evans TW. Bedside assessment of myocardial performance in the critically ill. *Int Care Med* 1994; **20**: 513–21.

Tobin M. *Principles and Practice of Intensive Care Monitoring*. McGraw Hill, 1998. New York

References

1. Artucio H, Pereira M. Cardiac arrhythmias in critically ill patients: Epidemiologic study. *Crit Care Med* 1990; **18**: 1383–8.

2. Pepine C. Prognostic markers in thrombolytic therapy: looking beyond mortality. *Am J Cardiol* 1996; **78**: 24–7.

3. Connors AF Jr, Speroff T, Dawson NV *et al*. The effectiveness of right heart catheterization in the initial care of critically ill patients. *J Am Med Assoc* 1996; **276**: 889–97.

4. Soni N. Swan song for the Swan–Ganz catheter? *Br Med J* 1996; **313**: 763–4.

6

RIGHT VENTRICLE

Despite its intimate connection with the LV and its important relationship with the lungs, ignorance of right ventricular function is widespread. There are reasons why such ignorance prevails:

- Early researchers had shown that if the pericardium is open and the right ventricular free wall was ablated by diathermy there were minimal effects on the haemodynamics.

- Replacing the free wall with a patch had little or no effect on the cardiac output or central venous pressures.[1]

- Furthermore, pioneers in paediatric cardiac surgery had shown that it was possible to bypass the RV altogether without affecting systemic venous pressures or compromising cardiac output.

These areas of research suggested:

- The RV was little more than a passive conduit of blood.

- Systemic venous pressures were high enough to drive blood through the low impedance pulmonary circuit to the LV.

Both these approaches had their flaws and it became clear over time that:

- If the pericardium was closed, damage to the free wall did affect the cardiac output adversely.

- That a persistent shunt in a child led eventually to systemic venous congestion.

- That such children could not pump blood through their lungs if the pulmonary vascular resistance rose for any reason.

It was now apparent that the RV was necessary for at least two reasons:

- To keep the systemic venous pressures low, particularly during exercise.

- To maintain flow through the lungs even if the vascular resistance should rise, as in disease states.

RIGHT VENTRICULAR ANATOMY AND PHYSIOLOGY

The widespread use of a two-dimensional, four-chamber view of the heart contributes to many of the misconceptions about the RV. Although it could not be described as inaccurate, it fails utterly to convey the differences between the two ventricles, an understanding of which is essential to its proper assessment and management.

There are important differences between the ventricles. The RV is:

- Thin walled unlike the thick wall of the LV.

- Crescentic in shape unlike the inverted bullet shape of the LV. This makes the RV less amenable to mathematical modelling. Consequently, it has proved more difficult to get any meaningful results from studies of the RV even with ultrasound.

- It wraps itself around the LV like an envelope lying largely anterior to it.

It is divided into:

- A heavily trabeculated inflow tract. The trabeculations in the inflow tract are said to improve mixing of the venous blood draining into the ventricle.

- An outflow tract which is less so.

- A completely smooth subpulmonic area.

- The interventricular septum that separates the two ventricles is very important in linking the function of the two ventricles but it should be considered an integral part of the LV.

Contraction develops in three phases:

- First, there is longitudinal shortening.

- The free wall moves towards the septum.

- Then contraction of the LV completes the ejection cycle like the wringing of a wet cloth.

Because of this complicated set of actions ejection from the RV is peristaltic and indeed a pressure gradient develops within the ventricle between the inflow and outflow tracts. The pressure generated is much less than in the LV, takes longer to develop and lasts longer. It is designed as a low pressure, volume displacement pump.[2]

The RV is supplied by the right coronary artery. It supplies:

- Most of the anterior wall.

- Lateral wall.

- Posterior third of the intraventricular septum.

Since the anterior two-thirds of the septum are supplied by the left coronary artery, it is not surprising that a variable area of the anterior wall adjacent to the septum is also supplied by the left coronary and can be involved in anterior infarctions.

The right coronary also supplies the posterior wall of the LV:

- In 50% of hearts. This is known as right sided dominance.

- In 25% the supply is shared between the two circulations (co-dominance).

- In 25% the left side is dominant.

The right coronary artery system drains not only eventually into the coronary sinus, but also directly into the right ventricular cavity via the thebesian veins.

When the right coronary is blocked an extensive collateral circulation can develop and supply the needs of the RV.

The RV is again different from the left because it is much more resistant to ischaemia. There are a number of reasons for this:

- Coronary flow can take place during systole and diastole because the pressure developed within the ventricle is less than the aortic pressure at all phases of the cardiac cycle.

- The RV functions as a low-pressure volume displacement pump and uses much less oxygen than the pressure work required of the LV.

- An extensive collateral circulation.

- Some of the oxygen requirements can be met by blood in the thebesian veins.

The RV, then, is a low-pressure volume displacement pump delivering blood to the pulmonary circulation. This has a very low impedance to ejection and the peak systolic pressure developed by the RV does not need to rise above 30 mmHg. Even during vigorous exercise when the cardiac output can rise to 30 litres/min there is minimal change in the systolic pressure generated. This is possible for three reasons:

- Recruitment of pulmonary capillaries to match the increase in flow.

- An increase in the calibre of the pulmonary capillaries.

- Increasing ventilation increases venous return.

Even under these conditions the systolic pressure in the pulmonary artery will stay below 40 mmHg.

Unlike the LV, the RV is very distensible and will increase in size readily if:

- It is overfilled.

- There is a sudden change in the impedance to ejection. The RV seems twice as sensitive to changes in ejection pressure as the LV.

The pericardium constrains this dilatation response, however, and if the reason for it persists then the septum is affected and it can be pushed over towards the LV. This will alter the compliance of the LV and can affect its output. The classic example of this is an acute pulmonary embolus. Not only is the filling of the LV impaired by obstruction to flow, but also the rapid right ventricular dilatation causes the septum to move across and impair the filling by reducing the left ventricular compliance. The consequence of this is a fall in cardiac output and a high left ventricular end-diastolic pressure (LVEDP) despite a normal LV.[3]

The interventricular septum is very important to the RV:

- It plays an important role in ejection

- It will sustain ejection from the RV even if the free wall is damaged.

- It helps to integrate the output from the two ventricles.

Another remarkable feature of the RV is its ability to adapt to adverse loading conditions. If the increase in filling is sustained, e.g. an atrial septal defect, or there is an sustained increase in the pulmonary vascular resistance as in chronic obstructive pulmonary disease, then the RV is capable of significant hypertrophy to the extent that it can eventually generate pressures as high as the left (it is also then much more likely to suffer ischaemia). Not only can it then sustain these high pressures, but also if it is unloaded by a lung transplant for example then it is capable of regressing back to its original state.[4]

Table 1 illustrates the level of pressure the adapted RV can achieve. It should be noted that in the group with very severe pulmonary hypertension the cardiac output failed to increase with exercise. Although the RV can generate the pressure, it may not maintain LV filling in pulmonary hypertension.

Conditions that might involve a normal ventricle include:

- Trauma.

- Myocardial infarction.

- Sepsis.

- Acute respiratory distress syndrome (ARDS).

Table 1 – Efects of exercise on the RV in various conditions. Adapted from data in ref. [2]

	RAP		RVP	
	Before	**After**	**Before**	**After**
CCF patients average PVRI 300	3	10	42	70
Rheumatic mitral valve patients average PRVI 482	6	8	46	87
Moderate pulmonary hypertension patients averrage PVRI 580	3	18	44	114
Severe pulmonary hypertension patients average PVRI 1480	5	13	85	147

- Post-cardiopulmonary bypass.
- Pulmonary embolus.
- Brain death.

Conditions that might involve an adapted ventricle include:

- Any of the above.
- Mitral valve disease.
- IPPV for exacerbation of COPD.
- Congestive cardiac failure.

The effect of a particular clinical circumstance will depend on the existing state of the RV. Are you dealing with a thin-walled volume displacement pump as in the sudden onset of ARDS in a young previously fit individual, or are you dealing with the same condition in a patient whose RV has already adapted to a chronic pressure overload? Clearly the approach to monitoring and supporting the RV should be different. The adapted ventricle is more robust and may need less support than the previously normal RV, which is easily compromised.

EMERGENCIES AFFECTING THE RV (SEE ALSO CHAPTER 4)

Trauma

Because of its anterior position the RV is very susceptible to myocardial contusion. There are many studies showing that it is common in chest injuries. In addition, there is some evidence that if RV contusion is present then both the morbidity and mortality rates from trauma are higher. The message is that such injuries are often overlooked and evidence of RV dysfunction should be sought and treated appropriately.

Even in the absence of direct trauma to the heart the RV is often under increased strain for two reasons:

- Contusion of the lungs often leads to an increase in the pulmonary vascular resistance. This means a rise in RV afterload.

- Hypotension can mean the RV blood supply is compromised. The development of ischaemia compromises the RV's ability to respond to acute changes in afterload.[5]

Myocardial infarction

Although an isolated RV infarction is possible it is very rare and involvement of the RV is much more common after an inferior infarction due to either occlusion of the circumflex or right coronary arteries. Because involvement of the RV worsens the prognosis of an inferior infarction evidence for it should be sought as revascularization by thrombolysis or angioplasty, if appropriate, improves the eventual outcome. Finding ST segment elevation in the right ventricular leads can make the diagnosis. V4R seems to be the most useful.

In the absence of additional ECG leads evidence of RV dysfunction can be sought by echocardiography. This may show:

- RV dilatation.

- Wall motion abnormalities.

- Paradoxical septal movement.

Damage will cause an impairment of compliance. There will be an increased resistance to filling early in diastole that worsens as the damaged RV follows its non-compliant pressure–volume curve. It then becomes very dependent on atrial contraction to augment its filling and maintain its stroke volume. Any deterioration in right atrial contractility, atrial arrhythmia or AV block will have a dramatic impact on stroke volume. In addition, a dilated RV shifts the interventricular septum towards the LV that can compromise left ventricular filling.[6]

As mentioned above, the anterior portion of the RV can also be involved in anterior myocardial infarctions if the septum is involved. Since septal contraction is very important in maintaining ejection from the RV and the left ventricular dysfunction associated with an anterior infarction may cause increased RV afterload it is not surprising that such infarcts may also be associated with RV dysfunction.

Acute respiratory distress syndrome (ARDS)

The multifactorial increase in the pulmonary vascular resistance and the compromising effects of positive pressure ventilation on RV filling are the main factors leading to RV compromise in this condition. Often the LV is functioning normally and it is the RV that needs monitoring and support.

Cardiopulmonary bypass

Although there are numerous causes of ventricular failure associated with cardiac surgery and cardiopulmonary bypass there are circumstances when the RV seems to be mostly affected. It is difficult to protect with cardioplegia as its anterior position means that it is susceptible to premature rewarming by the operating theatre lights. Venous blood returning to the right atrium is also responsible for some of this early rewarming. It is possible then to reach the end of a cardiac operation and find that the RV is stunned and performing poorly. Unfortunately one of the many consequences of cardiopulmonary bypass is an increase in the pulmonary vascular resistance. This increase in afterload can cause the dysfunctional RV to fail and prevent successful weaning from cardiopulmonary bypass.

Pulmonary embolus

This condition neatly illustrates the concept of ventricular interdependence. Since the outputs have to match it is clear that failure of one ventricle should affect the output of the other. The interventricular septum in this case seems to be important.

With a large pulmonary embolus:

- There is a dramatic rise in the impedance to ejection of the RV.

- This then dilates in response.

- The normally bowed septum flattens and moves into the left ventricular cavity.

- This raises the LVEDP although the actual filling of the LV has fallen and the cardiac output has dropped.

The drop in cardiac output may lead to a fall in the coronary perfusion pressure that may render the acutely overloaded RV ischaemic and lead to a worsening of the RV failure. This can lead eventually to RV infarction and death if not detected and treated.

RV dysfunction after pulmonary embolus also confers a worse prognosis and even in the normotensive patient signs of abnormal RV function should be sought.[3]

Brain death

Right ventricular failure after cardiac transplantation is a leading cause of morbidity and mortality. It has been attributed to an elevated pulmonary vascular resistance in the recipient. However, recent work has shown that the haemodynamic changes that occur as a consequence of brain death in the donor have a deleterious effect on ventricular function. The RV is more severely affected by these changes and cardiac preservation before transplantation causes a further decrease in RV function. It is now suggested that strategies to minimize RV dysfunction in the donor before harvesting should be employed to try and reduce early transplant morbidity and mortality rates.[7]

Mitral valve disease

The gradual increase in pulmonary venous pressure secondary to stenosis of the mitral valve leads to a rise in the pulmonary artery pressures. As this takes place slowly the RV has time to hypertrophy to cope with the increased afterload. It successfully maintains the flow despite having to generate pressures as high as in the systemic circulation. Eventually the flow starts to fall and the cardiac output drops. The systemic vascular resistance has to rise to maintain systemic pressure. In this situation any change in the delicate balance of afterload and coronary perfusion can have disastrous results.

Systemic sepsis is often responsible for a profound deterioration in these patients. The associated rise in pulmonary vascular resistance and the systemic hypotension which causes RV ischaemia cause a dramatic fall in RV output and there is a profound fall in BP because the capacity to increase the cardiac output in response to a drop in SVR is lost.

At this point the RV needs:

- Inotropic support to maintain its ejection.

- An increase in the coronary perfusion pressure to restore right coronary perfusion.

- Adrenaline may be beneficial because of its mixed α and β stimulant properties.

Although IPPV may increase afterload still further, its beneficial effects on oxygenation and its ability to lower CO_2 levels usually improves RV function and lowers the pulmonary vascular resistance.

Chronic obstructive pulmonary disease (COPD)

This disease leads to a gradual loss of the pulmonary vascular tree. As it is a slow process there is ample time for the RV to hypertrophy to maintain the pressures necessary to maintain flow through the lungs. However, during acute exacerbations the associated hypoxia and hypercapnia leads to myocardial ischaemia and an acute rise in the pulmonary vascular resistance. It must be remembered that there is often associated ischaemic heart disease. If positive pressure ventilation becomes necessary, this will add an increasing burden to an overloaded RV. Not only will it increase the afterload, but also it will compromise RV filling. Although the gradual improvement in hypercapnia and hypoxaemia will allow the RV to recover, it may need support during the acute phase of the illness.

Congestive cardiac failure

Chronic cardiac failure is the commonest cause of right heart failure. The chronic venous congestion creates a chronic pressure overload on the RV. The RV copes by chamber enlargement and hypertrophy. However, the LV must be considerably damaged before it affects the RV and it is suggested that its ejection fraction has to be < 30% for this to happen.[8]

DIAGNOSIS OF RV DYSFUNCTION

If one has a working knowledge of RV function, then clinical circumstances such as those outlined above should lead one to consider the possibility of RV dysfunction. Clinical features include:

- Raised CVP particularly if LV function normal.

- Tricuspid incompetence.

- Hepatomegaly and peripheral oedema.

There may be ECG changes of an inferior infarct. If there is right-sided dominance then posterior infarcts will involve the RV. Right ventricular leads such as V4R may show ischaemia.

Echocardiography will reveal abnormalities such as:

- Dilatation.

- Tricuspid incompetence.

- Abnormalities in wall motion.

- Paradoxical septal movement.

Use of the right ventricular ejection fraction PA catheter may show reduced EF or increased end-diastolic volumes. However, this catheter functions less well if there is tricuspid incompetence or fast atrial arrhythmias both of which are common in acute RV dysfunction and care should be exercised in interpreting the values obtained in the acutely ill patient.

Treatment of RV dysfunction

Attention must be paid to preload, afterload and contractility.

- The RV responds poorly to volume loading if the afterload is already high. For example, a pulmonary embolus will cause the RV to distend until it is constrained by the pericardium. Further filling will not help. Volume loading is only beneficial if the RV filling pressure is < 12 mmHg and the ventricle is not already constrained by the pericardium.

- Reducing the afterload means altering the pulmonary vascular resistance:

- Inhaled nitric oxide may be effective

- prostacyclin has been used, sometimes with noradrenaline to maintain systemic pressure

- However, if the blood flow through the lungs is so low that the cardiac output is compromised it may be that a high SVR is necessary to maintain coronary perfusion. Vasoconstrictors may be necessary to restore perfusion pressure to the right coronary before the RV will respond to inotropes.

For example, a patient with chronic mitral valve disease who becomes septic will be unable to increase their CO, the coronary perfusion pressure will drop and ischaemia will develop.

Noradrenaline may be necessary initially to stabilize this situation. Its benefits outweigh any effects it might have on the pulmonary circulation. Adrenaline is also useful because of its α effects on SVR and its β inotropic effects. There is no inotrope specific for the RV.

Further reading

Remetz MS, Cabin HS. The right ventricle. *Cardiol Clin* 1992; **10**: 1–196.

Rigolin VH, Robiolio PA, Wilson JS *et al*. The forgotten chamber: the importance of the right ventricle. *Cathet Cardiovasc Diagn* 1995; **35**: 18–28.

References

1. Kagan A. Dynamic responses of the right ventricle following extensive damage of cauterisation. *Circulation* 1952; **5**: 816.

2. Weber KT, Joseph JS, Schroff SG *et al*. The right ventricle: physiological and patho-physiological considerations. *Crit Care Med* 1983; **11**: 323–8.

3. Lualdi JC, Goldhaber SZ. Right ventricular dysfunction after acute pulmonary embolism: patho-physiologic factors, detection and therapeutic implications. *Am Heart J* 1995; **130**: 1276–82.

4. Moulton MJ, Creswell LL, Ungacta FF *et al*. Magnetic resonance imaging provides evidence for remodelling of the right ventricle after single lung transplantation for pulmonary hypertension. *Circulation* 1996; **94 (suppl.)**: II312–19.

5. Eddy CA, Rice CL. The right ventricle: An emerging concern in the multiply injured patient. *J Crit Care* 1989; **4**: 58–66.

6. Kinch JW, Ryan TJ. Right ventricular infarction. *N Engl J Med* 1994; **330**: 1211–17.

7. Bittner HB, Kendall SW, Chen EP, van Trigt P. The combined effects of brain death and cardiac graft preservation on cardiopulmonary haemodynamics and function before and after subsequent heart transplantation. *J Heart Lung Transplant (USA)* 1996; **15**: 764–77.

8. Boldt J, Zickmann B, Herold C *et al*. Right ventricular function in patients with reduced left ventricular function undergoing myocardial revascularization. *J Cardioth Vasc Anaesth* 1992; **6**: 24–8.

7

HEART AND CIRCULATION IN SEVERE SEPSIS

Sepsis is a common problem in clinical medicine either as the primary cause of admission or acquired (nosocomial) while in hospital.

A discussion of the heart and circulation in sepsis was thought appropriate for this text for several reasons:

- Physicians treat the cardiovascular effects of sepsis.

- Physicians are often asked to help manage patients with septic shock on surgical wards.

- It is important to appreciate the implications for management of sepsis-induced myocardial depression and failure.

This brief review is not intended to be a comprehensive account of pathophysiology, clinical features and therapy of sepsis (see further reading). Instead, the text concentrates on cardiovascular pathophysiology and its therapeutic implications.

DEFINITIONS

It is important that clinicians and researchers use the same definitions. A Consensus Conference[1] has proposed the following terminology:

- Infection – host response to the presence of microorganisms or tissue invasion by microorganisms.

- Bacteraemia – presence of viable bacteria in circulating blood.

- Sepsis – systemic response to infection. Defined as infection plus two or more of:

    Temperature > 38 or < 36°C
    Heart rate > 90 beats/min
    Respiratory rate > 20 beats/min or $p\mathrm{CO_2}$ < 4.3 kPa
    WCC > 12 000 or > 10% immature band forms

- Systemic inflammatory response syndrome (SIRS) – two or more of the above features of sepsis but in the absence of an infective cause. This recognizes that certain other pathological conditions can stimulate the body to respond in an identical fashion to that of infection, e.g. trauma, burns and pancreatitis. If SIRS or sepsis proceeds to severe sepsis or septic shock, the mortality rate increases.

- Severe sepsis – sepsis associated with organ dysfunction (e.g. oliguria) or hypotension but not requiring inotropic support or vasopressors.

- Septic shock – refers to the occurrence of shock in the presence of sepsis. This was defined as sepsis with hypotension not responding to fluid therapy and organ dysfunction or evidence of tissue hypoxia e.g. lactic acidosis. Owing to the significance of the development of shock from sepsis, it is septic shock that will mainly be discussing here.

The terms 'septicaemia' and 'sepsis syndrome' have been abandoned.

PROGNOSIS OF SEPTIC SHOCK

When sepsis progresses to septic shock there is a high mortality rate – about 40–80% depending on differing studies and rigour of definition. Poor outcome is associated with:

- Increased age.

- Degree of lactic acidaemia, i.e. degree of tissue hypoxia.

- Delay in antibiotic administration, or resistance developing.

- Immunosuppression, e.g. by chemotherapy or more commonly corticosteroids.

- Poor prognosis if immunoglobulin levels reduced or low WCC.

- Development of multiple organ failure and the number of organ systems failed.

CARDINAL PATHOPHYSIOLOGICAL CHANGES IN SEVERE SEPSIS

Myocardial depression

At first glance it seems a paradox to talk of myocardial depression in a condition frequently associated with a higher than normal cardiac output. However:

- Cardiac output is often partially maintained by tachycardia, i.e. stroke volume is reduced.

- There is depression of LV ejection fraction (LVEF). Both the LV and RV dilate once preload is restored.[2] Dilation may be an attempt to maintain stroke volume.

- In survivors the abnormality in LVEF is corrected by 7–10 days.

The decrease in myocardial function is due to:

- A circulating myocardial depressant factor.

- A relative circulatory resistance to catecholamines.

- Often, a fall in coronary perfusion pressure.

- In late stages a rise in pulmonary vascular resistance.

- *In vitro* studies also suggest a direct negative inotropic effect of nitric oxide.

Myocardial injury

A recent important study demonstrated significant increase in cardiac troponin I levels in patients with septic shock,[3] implying significant myocardial cell damage. (This is despite, in general, evidence of well-maintained coronary blood flow in septic shock.) Serum troponin levels tended to be lower in survivors than non-survivors and tended to be higher in patients on large doses of inotropes and vasopressors.

This study raises serious questions, at present unresolved:

- Is the reduction in cardiac function and cardiac dilation in septic shock related to myocardial depression or myocardial injury or both?

- Is the use of inotropes and vasopressors necessary because of the myocardial injury or a cause of myocardial injury by increasing myocardial oxygen requirements?

Vasodilation

- Nitric oxide – previously known as endothelium-derived relaxing factor (EDRF), is the principal mediator of vascular smooth muscle tone. Its release from vascular endothelium is the principal cause of the profound vasodilation seen in sepsis causing the characteristic fall in SVR. Nitric oxide is synthesized from the amino acid arginine by the action of nitric oxide synthase.

- Degree of vasodilation or peripheral vascular failure may be a major determinant of outcome. Cardiac output is generally well maintained, even elevated in response to the peripheral vasodilation.

- In severe cases the vasculature can lose its responsiveness to vasopressors.

Leaky capillaries

- Capillary endothelial damage results in increased vascular wall permeability, which leads to peripheral oedema. The leaky capillaries are **not** an indication for either fluid restriction or diuretics. Diuretics do not treat vascular damage.

Decreased circulating volume

- Vasodilation results in an expanded vascular space.

- Leaky capillaries contribute to this relative hypovolaemia.

- This is in addition to surgical fluid and blood losses in surgical sepsis and peritonitis

Hypotension

- From a combination of all of the above hypotension is produced. This would not be so bad in the face of a high flow from the elevated cardiac output if there was not an abnormal maldistribution of flow. For example, renal blood flow is impaired at an early stage.

Oxygen transport

- Oxygen consumption or VO_2 is reduced in septic shock often with evidence of tissue hypoxia, e.g. elevated blood lactate, often despite well-maintained cardiac output. In septic shock this may be due to maldistribution of blood flow, metabolic abnormalities, endothelial cell swelling or increased cellular membrane permeability.

- An inadequate VO_2 might suggest that global oxygen delivery is inadequate to maintain tissue oxygen needs. Some have taken the increase in lactate as evidence for **pathological supply dependency** (i.e. a straight-line relationship between tissue delivery and consumption over a wide range of values) and have promoted therapy to increase delivery (usually by increasing cardiac output). However, modern studies do not support widespread occurrence of oxygen supply dependency.

Clinical presentation

Classically septic shock has been subdivided into early 'warm' shock and late 'cold' shock with features as follows:

Warm shock:

- Hyperdynamic
- Warm skin
- Fever and chills
- Moderate hypotension
- Moderate urine output
- Bounding pulse
- Tachypnoea
- Low systemic vascular resistance
- High cardiac output
- Classically Gram-negative

Cold shock:

- Hypodynamic
- Cold and clammy
- Mottled skin
- Circulatory collapse
- Tachypnoea
- Oliguria
- Thready pulse
- High SVR
- Low cardiac output
- Classically Gram-positive

However, it is now recognized that there is no clear distinction in the clinical or haemodynamic profile of Gram-neagtive or -positive septic shock, i.e. the clinical features give no reliable clue to the nature of the infective organism. Although some patients may pass from a warm phase to a cold phase (especially if therapy is delayed), it is now recognized that the clinical features can be blurred with up to one-third of patients seemingly presenting with cold, low cardiac output shock with no prior hyperdynamic phase.[4]

DIAGNOSIS OF SEPTIC SHOCK

- Diagnosis is made on the above clinical and laboratory features especially in an appropriate setting for sepsis, e.g. following laparotomy or pneumonia.

- Cultures may not identify a causative organism (as few as 50% of patients with septic shock will have positive blood cultures). This should not necessarily reassure one that there is no organism! **Positive blood or other cultures are not necessary for the diagnosis to be made.**

- A strong index of suspicion is necessary especially in the immunosuppressed or patients on corticosteroids who may not show the usual clinical manifestations.

- In cases of acute collapse there will be no time to wait for the results of specific cultures, and empiric therapy including empiric choice of antibiotics is promptly required.

- Septic shock can mimic other conditions. Common sense should alert one to the possibility in an appropriate setting, e.g. following abdominal surgery.

- A common error is falsely to ascribe tachypnoea (a cardinal sign) to heart failure.

SEPTIC SHOCK THERAPY

Prevention

- Prevention may be easier than cure.

- Strict infection control procedures are crucial. The importance of regular hand washing by doctors cannot be overemphasized.

- Prophylactic antibiotics for certain surgical procedures are appropriate.

- Fever and suspected infection should be promptly investigated and treated.

Eradication of the infection

- Source of the sepsis must be promptly identified and appropriate antibiotics administered and surgical collections drained.

- Gram-negative bacterial lysis by antibiotics may be associated with a sudden release of endotoxin into the bloodstream ('fuelling the fire'). This should **not** limit the early administration of antibiotic therapy.

- IV catheters suspected of being colonized or infected must be removed and cultured.

- Liaison with microbiologists about local bacterial prevalence and sensitivities is an important factor in attempting to limit misuse of antibiotics. Antibiotic resistance is a major, ongoing problem and unnecessary use (especially of the wrong antibiotic) is a major factor in this. Ideally, the narrowest spectrum appropriate antibiotic should be used.

Supportive care

- General measures such as fluid therapy, nutritional support and IPPV if necessary must be applied as part of the general care of the critically ill patient.

- Managing the patient with septic shock in an ICU run by trained ICU specialists can improve survival rates.[5]

- Antibiotic therapy or cardiovascular support alone will provide disappointing results in the therapy of septic shock. Outcome is, perhaps obviously, improved when both are combined.

Neutralizing the effects of toxins, mediator blockade and experimental therapies

- It is suggested that haemofiltration may remove toxins and inflammatory mediators from the plasma, but at the moment this action is controversial.

- An early attempt to block the effect of endotoxin used the monoclonal antibody to endotoxin, centoxin. Despite initial encouraging results, disappointing results in controlled studies led to the commercial withdrawal of the compound.

- Interest at present, therefore, is more focussed on blocking the cytokine-mediated inflammatory cascade. Unfortunately, despite many studies and large financial investment, none have fulfilled their theoretical promise (see further reading).

- Historically, corticosteroids have been given in septic shock, but two large, controlled, multicentre studies from America have failed to demonstrate any beneficial effect. At present the administration of steroids in septic shock is not indicated.

- Attempts to block the excess effects of nitric oxide with analogues of arginine showed initial promise in case series, but later phase II trials were halted due to unexpected adverse events.

- All other experimental therapies (and many have been tried) remain just that, experimental.

CARDIOVASCULAR SUPPORT

Fluid therapy

- Fluids must be given to optimize preload as an initial step. However, it has been shown that some patients with septic shock show a diminished cardiovascular response to fluid loading – further evidence for the depressed cardiac function seen from sepsis. For example, a study has shown that similar increases in preload, as assessed with a pulmonary artery catheter, result in lesser increases in LV stroke work compared with 'control' critically ill patients without sepsis.[6]

- Fluid loading alone is unlikely to restore haemodynamic stability, especially if there is RV compromise. In some patients with septic shock, volume loading does not result in an increase in cardiac output because the RV fails perhaps due to pulmonary hypertension or reduced coronary perfusion pressure.

Thus, almost all patients will require cardiovascular support.

Goals of cardiovascular support

Early studies purported to show an improved survival when patients were treated to attain so-called 'optimal goals' found in survivors. These goals included supranormal amounts of cardiac index (> 4.5 l/min/m²), oxygen delivery and oxygen consumption. Unfortunately these studies were, in general, poorly controlled and non-randomized. More recent studies suggest that over aggressive inotropic support in an attempt to achieve these goals, often in elderly patients, results in a worse outcome[7] due to the development of myocardial ischaemia.

It would seem that it is the spontaneous **ability** (i.e. the cardiac reserve) of patients to generate these 'supranormal' cardiovascular values that is important for survival. Thus, it is not disputed that there are **survivors'** haemodynamic values. What is disputed is that one can improve survival in other patients by achieving these survivor values. Attempting to generate these high cardiac outputs is now seen as misplaced in many patients. Another pitfall would be to constrict the patient excessively – the goal is to reverse the abnormal vasodilation.

Thus, efforts should be directed towards restoring normal cardiac function and normal organ perfusion rather than supranormal values – especially in the elderly or in patients with pre-existing cardiac disease. A mean arterial pressure > 70 mmHg is especially important with regard to the kidneys, which lose their ability to autoregulate early in sepsis. Thus, what would otherwise seem to be a reasonable blood pressure may not be adequate to maintain renal function.

Inotropic and vasopressor support

If one remembers that the main abnormalities are myocardial depression and excessive vasodilation, one can predict the type of support required. From a practical point of view the choices come down to dopamine or adrenaline singly or noradrenaline and dobutamine in combination (Once output is satisfactory, perfusion pressure may be maintained by judicious use of noradrenaline.) Although still in some ways experimental, dopexamine deserves a special mention.

Note: Adrenaline and dopamine have vasopressor properties in addition to being positive inotropes with the pressor effects becoming increasingly predominant at higher doses. Some see this as an advantage (especially in America where dopamine has been commonly used as a single agent in septic shock, despite the limitations outlined below). Others see this as a problem as one cannot reliably assess their relative effects at a given dose without a pulmonary artery catheter and, more importantly, one cannot individually and solely titrate to either effect.

Dopamine

- An early choice for treatment of septic shock in many centres.

- However, in one study,[8] it was successful in restoring systemic haemo-dynamics in only 31% of septic patients. Noradrenaline was successful in 93%, and 10 of 11 patients who failed to respond to dopamine satis-factorily responded to noradrenaline.

- Another study[9] found that dopamine and noradrenaline both increased blood pressure but that dopamine had potentially adverse effects com-pared with noradrenaline on an index of splanchnic blood flow, gastric mucosal pH (pH_i).

- Dopamine is still widely used at low rates of infusion as an agent to pro-tect the kidney and to prevent renal failure. This is despite numerous editorials and review articles stating that it has **no** renal protective effect. Increases in urine output (which **are** common) are mainly due to its inotropic properties or direct diuretic effects.

- Dopamine's adverse effects are causing increasing concern and are lim-iting its use in many centres. The potential for causing tachycardia and arrhythmias has been known for a long time, but more recently it has become apparent that dopamine suppresses secretion of prolactin (even at so-called renal doses), which leads to a reduced cell-based immune response.[10]

Adrenaline (epinephrine)

- Early studies showed beneficial effects on systemic haemodynamics, e.g. increases in cardiac output, blood pressure, oxygen delivery and oxygen consumption.

- More recent studies have focussed on effects on metabolism, acid–base balance and splanchnic blood flow. On these counts there seem to be serious concerns about the use of adrenaline infusions, especially at the high doses often required in septic shock.

- For example, in a cross-over study[11] of adrenaline versus dobutamine/noradrenaline in combination, adrenaline was associated with increases in systemic and hepatic venous lactate and decreases in pH_i.

- Another study[12] found that dobutamine improved indices of gut perfusion when added to patients receiving adrenaline infusions, especially if gut perfusion was already impaired. This was achieved without an overall change in systemic haemodynamics.

- Additional adverse effects of adrenaline relate to its metabolic effects, i.e. increases blood sugar and lowers serum potassium.

Dobutamine

- Dobutamine[13] may be the inotropic agent of choice for optimizing cardiac output (and therefore global organ blood flow) in septic shock. Cardiac output will increase, but those patients requiring vasopressor support may require an increased rate of infusion.

- Dobutamine has inconsistent effects on indices of splanchnic blood flow. Excessive rates of infusion may be detrimental[7] presumably by increasing myocardial oxygen demand and causing ischaemia. This is probably only a problem in elderly patients with concomitant ischaemic heart disease.

Note: Myocardial depression of sepsis is reversible whereas ischaemic heart disease is not.

Noradrenaline (norepinephrine)

- As stated above, noradrenaline increases blood pressure more reliably than dopamine.

- Increase in pressure increases coronary perfusion pressure with, for example, improvements in RV function.

- Unlike dopamine there are many studies showing increases in urine output and creatinine clearance when noradrenaline is administered in septic shock. For example, when noradrenaline was added to a regimen of fluids, dopamine and/or dobutamine, there were further increases in blood pressure and significant increases in creatinine clearance.[14]

- Despite its vasoconstrictor properties, noradrenaline may increase indices of splanchnic blood flow in septic shock.[15]

- Why should noradrenaline, a vasoconstrictor, seemingly have a more beneficial effect on splanchnic blood flow than adrenaline, another vasoconstrictor? One theory is that it relates to the different ways they may be used. Noradrenaline is often used in combination with dobutamine and its effects are titrated to reverse the abnormal degree of vasodilation while, hopefully avoiding actual vasoconstriction. Adrenaline, however, if used as a sole agent, cannot control in the same way its potential to cause actual vasoconstriction.

- Although not ideal practice, if one has to administer vaso-active agents 'blind', i.e. in the absence of invasive monitoring on a ward, then noradrenaline is arguably the best agent for this purpose in septic shock.

- Use of noradrenaline should be cautious as excessive vasoconstriction may occur especially if the patient is hypovolaemic.

- A commonly expressed fear is that use of noradrenaline may cause falls in cardiac output as a response to increases in afterload. In fact, adding noradrenaline to patients resistant to dobutamine commonly causes **increases** in cardiac output.[16]

Phenlyephrine is a pure vasoconstrictor. It is occasionally effective where noradrenaline has failed.

Dopexamine

- Dopexamine is a relatively new drug with predominantly β_2-stimulating properties, i.e. it is a potent inotrope and vasodilator causing only minor increases in myocardial oxygen consumption and negligible arrhythmias. In addition, dopexamine has significant dopaminergic stimulant activity.

- Recent concerns over 'renal dose dopamine' to preserve renal function have encouraged some centres increasingly to use dopexamine for this purpose with some initial encouraging results.

- Splanchnic blood flow is increased with dopexamine, increased pH_i may be normalized and indices of gastrointestinal permeability reduced. The significance of these with regard to outcome is currently unclear.

- The most interesting aspect of dopexamine and the most controversial is the suggestion that it may have specific anti-inflammatory properties.[17] Most of the evidence for this to date is from animal studies, but a few studies on surgical patients broadly support the hypothesis. Further evidence is eagerly awaited.

SUMMARY OF CARDIOVASCULAR SUPPORT

- Dobutamine is probably still the positive inotrope of choice in sepsis.

- There should be a limited role for dopamine despite its often beneficial haemodynamic effects, partly because there are better agents available, but mainly due to increasing concern over adverse effects.

- Noradrenaline is the vasopressor of choice.

- Adverse effects of adrenaline should limit its use to emergency resuscitation.

- The combination of fluid therapy, dobutamine and noradrenaline has much to commend it and is the standard approach in many centres.

- There may be an increasing role for dopexamine, especially if specific anti-inflammatory effects are substantiated.

Further reading

Grocott-Mason RM, Shah AM. Cardiac dysfunction in sepsis: new theories and clinical implications. *Int Care Med* 1998; **24**: 286–95.

Parrillo JE. Pathogenetic mechanisms of septic shock. *N Engl J Med* 1993; **328**: 1471–7.

Task Force of the American College of Critical Care Medicine, Society of Critical Care Medicine. Practice parameters for haemodynamic support of sepsis in adult patients in sepsis. *Crit Care Med* 1999; **27**: 639–60.

Zeni F, Freeman B, Natanson C. Anti-inflammatory therapies to treat sepsis and septic shock: a reassessment. *Crit Care Med* 1997; **25**: 1095–1100.

References

1. American College of Chest Physicians/Society of Critical Care Medicine Consensus Conference. Definitions for sepsis and organ failure and guidelines for the use of innovative therapies in sepsis. *Crit Care Med* 1992; **20**: 864–74.

2. Parker MM, McCarthy KE, Ognibene FP, Parrillo JE. Right ventricular dysfunction and dilatation, similar to left ventricular changes, characterise the cardiac depression of septic shock in humans. *Chest* 1990; **97**: 126–31.

3. Turner A, Tsamitros M, Bellomo R. Myocardial cell injury in septic shock. *Crit Care Med* 1999; **27**: 1775–80.

4. Jardin F, Brun-Ney D, Auvert B, Beauchet A, Bourdarias JP. Sepsis-related cardiogenic shock. *Crit Care Med* 1990; **18**: 1055–60.

5. Reynolds HN, Haupt MT, Thill-Baharozian MC, Carlson RW. Impact of critical care physician staffing on patients with septic shock in a university hospital medical intensive care unit. *J Am Med Assoc* 1988; **260**: 3446–50.

6. Ognibene FP, Parker MM, Natanson CC, Shelhamer JH, Parrillo JE. Depressed left ventricular performance. Response to volume infusion in patients with sepsis and septic shock. *Chest* 1988; **93**: 903–10.

7. Hayes MA, Timmins AC, Yau EH *et al*. Elevation of systemic oxygen delivery in the treatment of critically ill patients. *N Engl J Med* 1994; **330**: 1717–22.

8. Martin C, Papazian L, Perrin G *et al*. Norepinephrine or dopamine for the treatment of hyperdynamic septic shock? *Chest* 1994; **103**: 1826–31.

9. Marik PE, Mohedin M. The contrasting effects of dopamine and norepinephrine on systemic and splanchnic oxygen utilisation in hyperdynamic sepsis. *J Am Med Assoc* 1994; **272**: 1354–7.

10. Bailey AR, Burchett KR. Effect of low dose dopamine on serum concentrations of prolactin in critically ill patients. *Br J Anaesth* 1997; **78**: 97–9.

11. Meier-Hellmann A, Reinhart K, Bredle DL *et al*. Epinephrine impairs splanchnic perfusion in septic shock. *Crit Care Med* 1997; **25**: 399–404.

12. Levy B, Bollaert PE, Luchelli JP *et al*. Dobutamine improves the adequacy of gastric mucosal perfusion in epinephrine-treated septic shock. *Crit Care Med* 1997; **25**: 1649–54.

13. Vincent JL, Roman A, Kahn RJ. Dobutamine administration in septic shock: addition to a standard protocol. *Crit Care Med* 1990; **18**: 689–93.

14. Redl-Wenzl EM, Armbruster C, Edelmann G *et al*. The effects of norepinephrine on hemodynamics and renal function in severe septic shock states. *Int Care Med* 1993; **19**: 151–4.

15. Meier-Hellmann A, Specht M, Hannemann L *et al*. Splanchnic blood flow is greater in septic shock treated with norepinephrine than in severe sepsis. *Int Care Med* 1996; **22**: 1354–9.

16. Martin C, Viviand X, Arnaud S *et al*. Effects of norepinephrine plus dobutamine or norepinephrine alone on left ventricular performance of septic shock patients. *Crit Care Med* 1999; **7**: 1708–13.

17. Byers RJ, Eddleston J, Pearson RC *et al*. Dopexamine reduces the incidence of acute inflammation in the gut mucosa after abdominal surgery in high risk patients. *Crit Care Med* 1999; **27**: 1787–93.

8

ECHOCARDIOGRAPHY AND CARDIAC EMERGENCIES

Echocardiography is an important basic investigation in the management of cardiac emergencies. It provides useful information about cardiac structure and function to aid diagnosis and risk stratification. However, like all imaging modalities, it has both advantages and limitations. It is important to remember these limitations and treat the patient, not the echocardiogram, and to seek alternative strategies when appropriate or when clinical findings fail to tally with echocardiographic findings.

This chapter will discuss the uses, advantages and limitations of, indications for and alternatives to transthoracic and transoesophageal echo, and explain how to interpret the echo report, in general and in relation to each of the common cardiac emergencies.

Abbreviations used:

- TTE – transthoracic echocardiogram.
- TOE – transoesophageal echocardiogram.
- CT – computed tomography.
- MRI – magnetic resonance imaging.
- LA – left atrium.
- RA – right atrium.
- LV – left ventricle.
- RV – right ventricle.
- EF – ejection fraction.
- FS – fractional shortening.
- AS – aortic stenosis.

- MS – mitral stenosis.
- EOA – effective orifice area.
- AVG – aortic valve gradient.
- MVG – mitral valve gradient.
- TVG – tricuspid valve gradient.
- AR – aortic regurgitation.
- MR – mitral regurgitation.
- TR – tricuspid regurgitation.
- ASD – atrial septal defect.
- VSD – ventricular septal defect.

TRANSTHORACIC ECHOCARDIOGRAM (TTE)

Uses

Provides diagnostic information about structural abnormalities and their functional significance. TTE is useful for the assessment of:

- Atrial and ventricular size, shape and function.
- Myocardial thickness.
- Valve structure and function.
- Aortic root.
- Pericardial effusions.
- Intracardiac masses.
- Congenital and acquired heart defects, and connections between great vessels and the heart.
- In babies and small children, ascending aorta, aortic arch, proximal descending aorta and pulmonary artery up to the bifurcation may also be well visualized.
- Pulmonary artery pressure (may be estimated in the presence of tricuspid regurgitation and absence of pulmonary stenosis).

Advantages

- Portable – can bring equipment to sick patient rather than move patient to test facility.

- Does not limit access to sick patient for clinician, nurse or monitoring equipment.

- Can be performed in upright position in severely orthopnoeic patients.

- Non-invasive and safe – therefore also highly suitable as follow-up investigation.

- Relatively cheap.

- Widely available.

Limitations

- Image quality is dependent on operator skills, patient anatomy and position. Generally best in left lateral position. May be severely impaired by air between chest wall and heart, e.g. hyperinflated lungs in obstructive airways disease, patients on mechanical ventilator, pneumothorax, supine or right lateral position. Narrow rib spaces and obesity may also cause technical difficulty.

- Information is often qualitative rather than quantitative. Significant intra- and inter-observer variation when images suboptimal.

- Left atrial appendage and in adults, superior vena cava and majority of aorta and pulmonary arteries above valve/root level, cannot be imaged.

- Image quality generally inferior to transoesophageal echo.

- Limited capacity for differentiation between different types of tissues and fluids.

TRANSOESOPHAGEAL ECHOCARDIOGRAM (TOE)

Uses

- Like TTE, provides diagnostic information about structural abnormalities and their functional significance.

- Image quality better than TTE. Particularly useful when better resolution of detail is needed.

prosthetic valve dysfunction

- endocarditis (e.g. on valves, central venous lines, pacing leads) and its complications (e.g. annular abscess, fistulae)

- atrial septal defects (ASD)

- atrial masses

- inadequate TTE

- strong suspicion of cardiac pathology despite negative TTE

- Can also image additional structures not imaged by TTE:

    thoracic aorta, e.g. in aortic dissection/transection

    left atrial appendage, e.g. cardiac source of thromboemboli

    pulmonary artery up to the bifurcation

    superior vena cava

- Complements TTE; does not replace it. Rarely, if ever, indicated without prior TTE – unlike good TTE, views are often off-axis, reducing accuracy of assessment of chamber dimensions, myocardial thickness, left ventricular function, Doppler flow velocities and valve gradients (often underestimated).

Advantages

- Portable – can bring equipment to sick patient rather than move patient to test facility. Can be performed intra-operatively.

- Does not limit access to sick patient for clinician, nurse or monitoring equipment.

- Low risk procedure in patients who are relatively well.

- Relatively cheap.

- Image quality relatively independent of patient anatomy and position.

Limitations

- Most centres perform TOE under sedation due to patient intolerance of associated discomfort, or general anaesthesia in patients at high risk with sedation.

- Semi-invasive – risks low but potentially severe: regurgitation/vomiting with aspiration, oesophageal perforation in oesophageal pouch or abnormal oesophagus (e.g. neoplasia), bacteraemia.

- Information is often qualitative rather than quantitative.

- Limited capacity for differentiation between different types of tissues and fluids.

- Not possible to image section of aortic arch where it crosses left main bronchus due to interference from air/bronchus interface.

- Inferobasal wall and true apex sometimes difficult to image satisfactorily.

Requirements for TOE under sedation

- Patient fit for sedation – commonly used sedative: benzodiazepine, e.g. IV midazolam or diazepam. If not, need to consider TOE under general anaesthesia.

- Able to lie flat in left lateral position.

- Patient fasted for at least 4 h.

- Information about medications, drug abuse, alcohol excess, allergies. May interfere with ease of sedation. May require antibiotic prophylaxis (similar to simple gastroscopy) in high-risk patients (e.g. previous or suspected endocarditis, prosthetic valves).

- Suitable for blind oesophageal intubation. Oesophageal perforation unlikely – no significant dysphagia, no known oesophageal pouch or friable oesophageal wall (e.g. neoplasm). No major maxillofacial trauma.

- Intra-procedural safety measures available – oxygen, suction, monitoring (ECG, pulse, blood pressure, oxygen saturation), qualified assistant (preferably two).

- Suitable after-care till patient sufficiently awake. Avoid food or drink for 2 h after procedure if pharyngeal local anaesthetic spray used as control of swallowing may be affected.

COMMON INDICATIONS FOR ECHOCARDIOGRAPHY

Myocardial infarction

Especially if new murmurs, intractable heart failure and/or hypotension not obviously due to severe continuing ischaemia (chest pain, ECG changes).

- Echo may demonstrate impaired function in both ventricles but not their relative haemodynamic contributions. Clinical/ECG/chest X-ray assessment and pulmonary artery catheter pressure measurements may be more useful than echo in distinguishing between hypotension due to poor left ventricular function and hypotension due to acute right ventricular infarction.

- May have complications of post-infarct ventricular septal defect (figure 1), ruptured papillary muscle with severe acute mitral regurgitation,

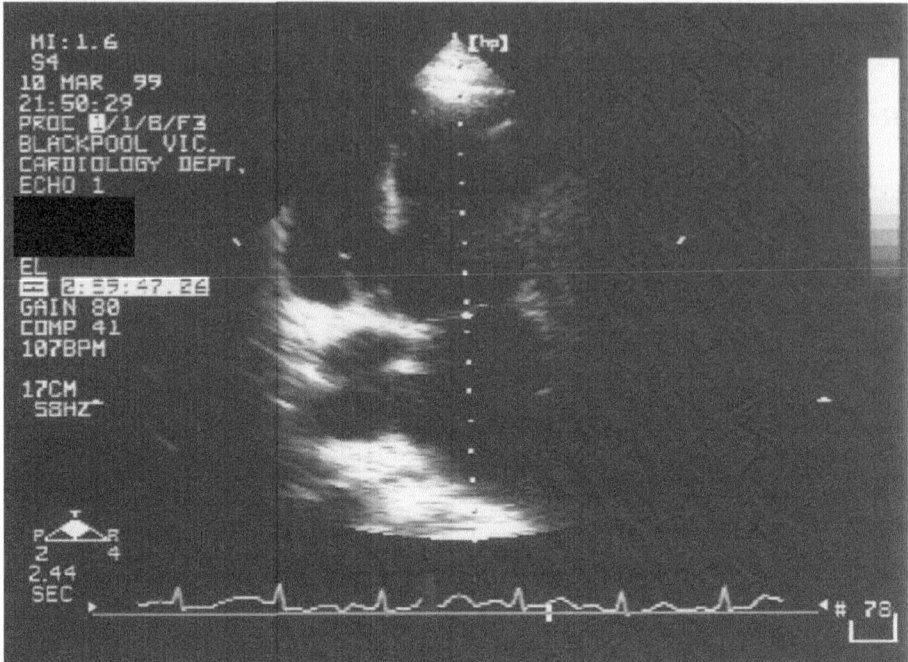

Figure 1 – TTE. Apical four-chamber view demonstrating a post-infract VSD.

rarely myocardial rupture with subacute cardiac tamponade (most arrest suddenly and die before investigation).

- Echo LVEF is calculated from linear measurements using the basic assumption of a truncated symmetrical ellipsoid shape. Substantial inaccuracies arise if images are suboptimal, resulting in errors subsequently magnified by multiplication during calculation, and/or if LV is asymmetrically impaired by regional myocardial infarction, when the basic assumptions about LV shape used in calculation no longer hold true.

- Subjective estimates by an experienced echocardiographer may be preferable. Moderate LV dysfunction generally equates to LVEF 30–40% (normal $\geq$ 50%). Qualitative echo assessment of LV contractility can be as effective as calculated LVEF in selecting patients who will benefit from ACE inhibitors (TRACE trial, wall motion index scoring).[1]

- LVEF is a load-dependent parameter and varies with prevailing haemodynamic conditions.

Note: should not rely heavily on LVEF alone as the indicator of LV dysfunction

- Other features are also very important. Large complete Q wave infarcts on ECG, especially anterior infarcts, widespread loss of R wave on ECG, large cardiac enzyme rises and clinical or radiographic heart failure all suggest need for ACE inhibitors, probably even if calculated LVEF does not meet trial criteria (e.g. big anterior infarct with echo LVEF 45%). Anterior infarction is also associated with higher incidence of LV thrombus (11%) than other sites (2%).

- MUGA radionuclide left ventriculography was used in SOLVD and SAVE trials. MUGA LVEF measurements are more reliable and reproducible than echo in the unselected population, but are still subject to 5–10% variation, are more time-consuming and costly, and involve radiation. Echo is usually adequate to guide clinical decisions.

- Anticoagulation[2] should be considered regardless of whether in sinus rhythm or atrial fibrillation to reduce stroke (SAVE trial) and cardiac mortality (SOLVD trial). Poor LV function is sufficient indication for anticoagulation[3] without demonstration of LV thrombus (figure 2).

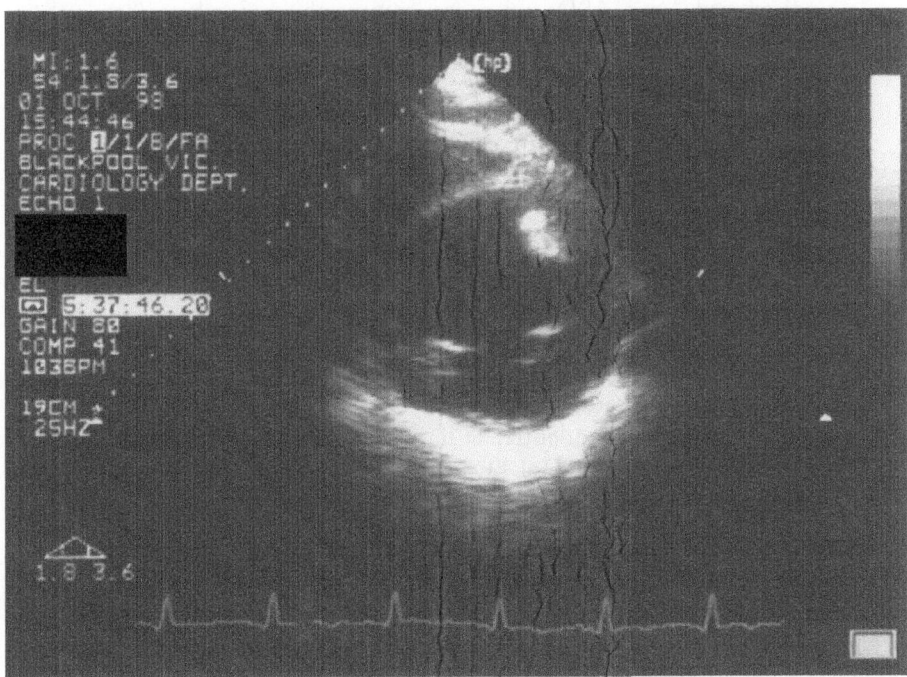

Figure 2 – TTE. Sagittal view of LV Mural thrombus.

Pulmonary oedema: heart failure

- Echo is particularly useful for diagnosis of significant systolic LV dysfunction, valve disease, dilated and hypertrophic cardiomyopathies. Mitral and aortic valve disease are commonest; isolated tricuspid disease the rarest. If TTE fails to confirm strong clinical suspicion of severe valve disease, especially prosthetic valve dysfunction, consider TOE.

- Diastolic LV dysfunction is difficult to assess. LV hypertrophy is a clue to hypertensive heart failure with preserved systolic function but diagnosis remains clinical.

- Pericardial constriction and restrictive cardiomyopathy are difficult to diagnose on echo. There may be no specific features. LV may appear mildly impaired. Pericardium is often echobright even when normal, and changes in thickness and calcification are often not detectable. Suspicion must be clinical (e.g. oedema out of proportion to degree of LV dysfunction) and confirmation of diagnosis sought by other means – cardiac catheter studies for intracardiac pressures, myocardial biopsy for amyloid, computed tomography (CT) or magnetic resonance imaging (MRI) for pericardial thickening and/or calcification.

- Isolated right heart failure may be primarily cardiac (e.g. previously undiagnosed large ASD) or more commonly, secondary (cor pulmonale, pulmonary embolism, rarely primary pulmonary hypertension). Right atrial and ventricular dilatation, tricuspid regurgitation and raised pulmonary pressures are the main echo findings. ASD may not be well imaged on TTE and may require TOE to confirm diagnosis and assess suitability for percutaneous device closure.

Endocarditis

- Main functions of echo are confirmation of diagnosis by demonstration of vegetations (figure 3), and assessment of extent and severity of infection and complications.

- TTE may be adequate to provide the diagnosis but is much less sensitive than TOE. Consequently, TOE has become a routine investigation for endocarditis, including TTE-proven endocarditis, and especially for prosthetic valve endocarditis.

- Extent of infection – number of valves affected, extent of valve infection, involvement of adjacent structures. Helps surgeon plan operation (e.g. mitral valve inspection as well as replacement of damaged aortic valve, mitral valve repair rather than replacement).

- Complications – severe valvular regurgitation. Annular abscess – may rupture to communicate with the circulation, become aneurysmal, form

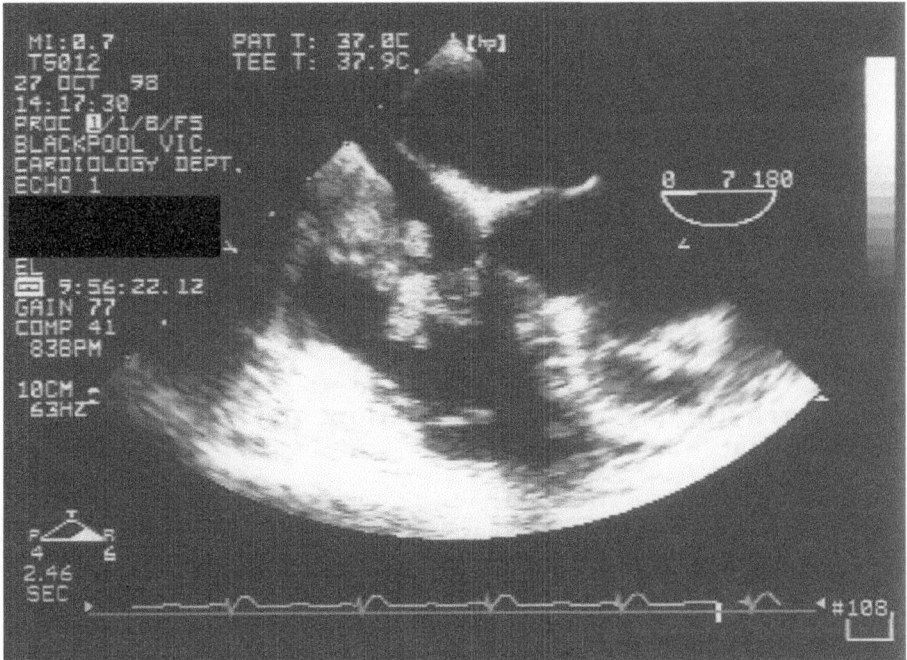

Figure 3 – TOE of endocarditis with large vegetation on pacing lead.

fistulae or rupture into pericardial space to cause haemopericardium and sudden death. Emboli.

- Echocardiographic indications for early surgery before completion of 6-week course of antibiotic therapy include worsening valvular regurgitation and enlarging abscesses which suggest failure of antibiotic therapy, unstable 'rocking' prosthetic valves at risk of complete dehiscence, and large and expanding aneurysms at high risk of rupture. There is some evidence that vegetations > 10 mm diameter have high risk of embolization but no conclusive evidence that surgery is indicated based on vegetation size alone.

Note: echo can never 100% exclude or confirm endocarditis. Vegetations may be too small to visualize. May be impossible to differentiate between new vegetations, old healed vegetations, thrombus (e.g. on pacing lead or prosthetic valve), calcific masses on degenerate valves and rare valve tumours. Diagnosis is ultimately clinical, albeit aided by echo.

Exertional syncope: ventricular arrhythmias

- Echo may be normal in ischaemic heart disease or show previous infarction, regional LV dysfunction or LV aneurysm formation.

- LV dysfunction is often global in dilated cardiomyopathies.

- Hypertrophic cardiomyopathy and aortic stenosis should be excluded by echo before provocative stress testing for malignant arrhythmias in patients with marked ECG changes of LV hypertrophy or suggestive clinical signs.

- Arrhythmogenic right ventricular dysplasia may be widespread with isolated RV dysfunction or localized/patchy with normal echo appearances.

- Echo is usually normal in right ventricular outflow tract ventricular tachycardia.

Atrial arrhythmias – atrial fibrillation, atrial flutter, atrial tachycardia

- Unexplained atrial arrhythmias may be the initial presenting feature of ischaemic heart disease, cardiomyopathy, valve disease especially mitral, and ASD.

- Atrial fibrillation and flutter predispose to left atrial (LA) thrombus and systemic thromboembolism.[4] Thrombo-embolic risks are reduced by adjusted-dose anticoagulation to an INR = 2.0–3.0. Risks are low (0.5% p.a.) in patients < 65 years with lone atrial fibrillation, similar to sinus rhythm (0.3% p.a.) and do not warrant anticoagulation.

Presence of clinical:

- past embolus

- heart failure

- hypertension

- diabetes mellitus

- atherosclerosis – coronary, peripheral or cerebrovascular

- and possibly age

and echocardiographic:

- TTE or TOE:

- LA diameter > 5 cm

- LV dysfunction

- LA or LV thrombus

- mitral stenosis

- mitral annular calcification

- TOE – dense LA or LV spontaneous echo contrast (implies sluggish blood flow)
- LA appendage thrombus
- low LA appendage peak flow velocities $\leq$ 20 cm/s
- complex aortic atheroma

risk factors are indications for anticoagulation. Clinical and TTE assessment are generally adequate to determine need for anticoagulation. TOE is not required routinely.

- Early DC cardioversion without $\geq$ 3 weeks of adequate prior anticoagulation may be preferable but not essential on clinical grounds. TOE may be used to exclude intracardiac thrombus before cardioversion.[5] TTE alone is inadequate (cannot image LA appendage). Note: exclusion of thrombus by echo does not obviate the need for peri- and post-cardioversion anticoagulation for atrial stunning.

Pericardial tamponade

- Pericardial tamponade is a clinical diagnosis.
- Echo can only diagnose a pericardial fluid collection (figure 4), demonstrate its size, distribution and suitability for safe pericardiocentesis via

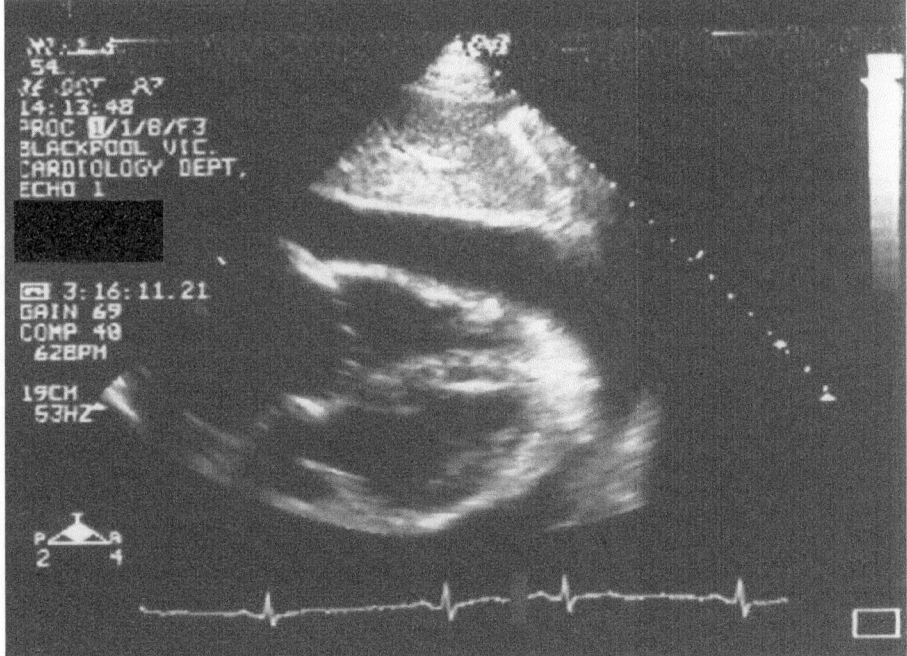

Figure 4 – TTE. Sub-costal view of pericardial effusion.

the subxiphisternal route, and provide evidence of haemodynamic effects but not their clinical significance. Right atrial and RV outflow tract diastolic collapse are non-specific and common even without clinical tamponade. Dilated inferior vena cava > 2 cm with > 50% inspiratory collapse, extensive RV collapse and > 40% inspiratory fall in early mitral inflow velocity suggest significant tamponade but may not always be present.

Major pulmonary embolism

- Diagnosis is largely clinical.

- Echo findings of RV dilatation/dysfunction and pulmonary hypertension with small/normal LV support the diagnosis but are not diagnostic. Diagnostic findings of mobile right heart thrombus or saddle embolus at the pulmonary bifurcation are rare and may require TOE.

Major chest trauma[6]

- Penetrating injury – echo finding of pericardial fluid collection suggests possible injury to the heart and warrants urgent surgical exploration.

- Blunt trauma and deceleration injuries, e.g. in road traffic accidents. The heart may hit the anterior chest wall resulting in myocardial contusions or anterior myocardial infarction due to trauma to left anterior descending artery. Distortion of the heart may result in valve leaflet or chordal rupture and significant valvular regurgitation. Descending aorta is relatively immobile and sudden shift of heart and aortic arch with sudden deceleration may result in aortic transection/rupture.

- TTE should be considered in all patients with major chest trauma. TOE is warranted where cardiac injury is suspected but TTE images inadequate (often the case in supine ventilated patients) and also where aortic injury is possible, unless alternative imaging modalities are used. TOE is frequently preferred to CT or MRI because it can be performed on the intensive care unit. There may be no murmurs with gross valvular regurgitation if flow is free and non-turbulent. LV contusions may be associated with only minor non-specific T-wave changes. Aortic transections may be silent initially, contained by haematoma with little bleeding and normal mediastinum on chest X-ray, but carry risk of acute rupture and sudden death.

Aortic dissection

- TTE may confirm diagnosis only if dissection involves the aortic root as ascending aorta and arch are usually poorly seen in adults. It may show the aortic dissection flap and possible complications – aortic valve involvement, aortic regurgitation, pericardial fluid collection (possible haemopericardium), cardiac tamponade, regional LV dysfunction or akinesia from coronary artery occlusion.

- Note: negative TTE does not exclude aortic dissection. Further investigation is necessary. TOE, dynamic contrast spiral CT, MRI and aortic angiography all have $\geq$ 95% sensitivity and specificity. TOE (figure 5) is frequently preferred in acute dissection as it can be performed on the intensive care unit. It will satisfactorily differentiate between dissections involving (Type A, emergency surgery is indicated) and not involving (Type B, conservative management if complications absent) the ascending aorta and identify the entry site for the surgeon. If complications involving the abdominal aorta are present (e.g. ischaemic leg), CT or MRI may be preferable as a single investigation that can also image the abdominal aorta as well. Current MRI scanners still limit access to patients, may interfere with monitoring and therapeutic equipment, and are more often used for chronic dissections and follow-up. Aortic angiography is generally not available in district general hospitals, carries an appreciable risk of catheter-related vascular damage, but can be combined with coronary angiography and might therefore be the

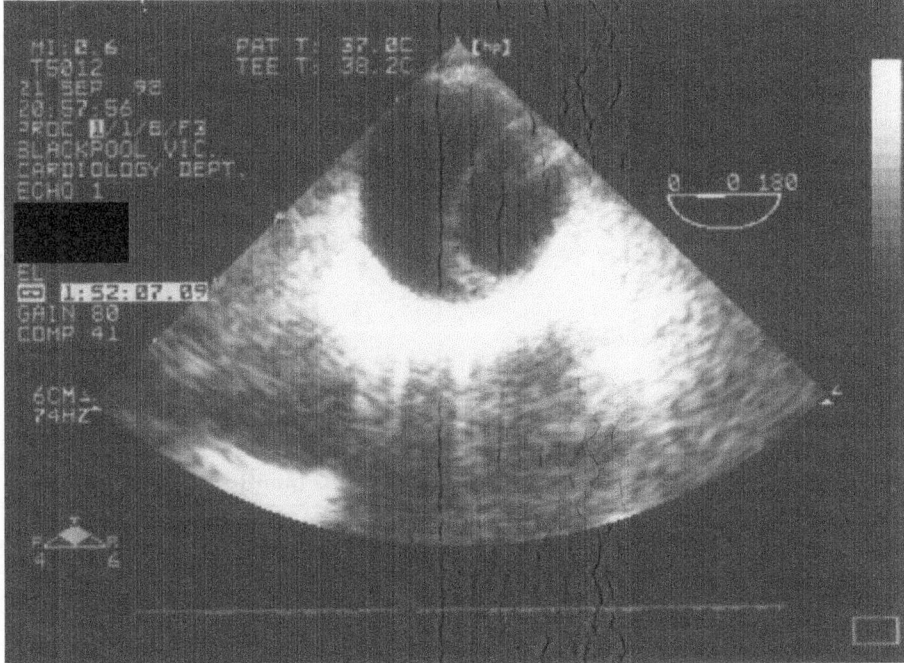

Figure 5 – TOE of type B aortic dissection.

technique of choice if concomitant severe ischaemic heart disease is suspected.

Interpretation of echo reports

Normal values

- LA diameter – 3–4 cm

- LV internal diameter – diastole 3.5–5.9 cm, systole 2.4–4.0 cm

- LV thickness:

    septum – 0.8–1.3 cm males, 0.7–1.0 cm females

    posterior wall – 0.8–1.1 cm males, 0.6–1.1 cm females

- LVEF – $\geq$ 50% (higher with severe MR/AR)

- FS – 28–44%

Systolic heart failure

Likely if:

- EF < 40%

- FS < 20%

- LV end systolic volume > 70 ml

- Extensive regional wall dysfunction

- Moderate-to-severe reduction in contractility

Possibly if:

- EF – 40–50%

- FS – 20–25%

Aortic stenosis (AS)

	Peak AVG (mmHg)	Mean AVG (mmHg)	EOA (cm^2)
Mild	15–30	<20	
Moderate	31–50	20–30	>1.0
Moderately severe	50–60	30–40	0.75–1.0
Severe	>60	>40	<0.75

Moderately severe and severe AS are haemodynamically significant and may warrant further investigation with a view to valve replacement.

- With poor LV function, valve gradient may be low and severity of stenosis underestimated. Low LV systolic pressures may result in peak AVG of only 30–40 mmHg despite severe AS. EOA by the continuity equation is a more accurate measure of severity in this situation.

Mitral stenosis

	EOA (cm²)	Pressure half-time (ms)	Mean MVG (mmHg)
Mild	1.5–2.0	< 150	< 5
Moderate	1.0–1.5	150–200	5–10
Severe	< 1.0	> 200	> 10

- Echo findings of dilated right heart, impaired RV and pulmonary hypertension are indications for intervention even if relatively asymptomatic.

- Criteria for percutaneous valvotomy are:

    thickening confined mainly to leaflet tips; mobile anterior leaflet

    little chordal involvement

    no commissural calcification

    at most mild mitral regurgitation

    no LA thrombus (need TOE to rule out LA and LA appendage thrombus)

Aortic (AR) and mitral (MR) regurgitation

- AR and MR are assessed by width and depth of regurgitant jet on colour flow Doppler, strength and duration of pulsed wave Doppler signal in relation to distance from regurgitant valve, strength and duration of continuous wave Doppler signal. Pressure half-time is also useful in AR – AR is usually haemodynamically significant if pressure half-time < 400 ms. Severity of AR and MR may be underestimated if regurgitant jets are eccentric and difficult to image. If TTE findings do not tally with clinical findings of severe regurgitation, consider TOE.

- Severity is usually graded out of 4 and expressed as:

    Grade 1/4 or grade 1+ or mild regurgitation

    Grade 2/4 or grade 2+ or moderate regurgitation

    Grade 3/4 or grade 3+ or moderately severe regurgitation

    Grade 4/4 or grade 4+ or severe regurgitation

- Grades 3 (moderately severe) and 4 (severe) are haemodynamically significant and warrant assessment by a cardiologist. Surgery should be considered if there are clinical sequelae (breathlessness, heart failure) or features of deteriorating cardiac function (dilated LV, impaired LV contractility, and particularly with MR, pulmonary hypertension).

- Trivial or mild AR and MR are common as physiological regurgitation is increasing being detected with the aid of improved technology in normal people. In general, if the valve appears normal and there is no murmur, antibiotic prophylaxis is unnecessary.

- Mild-to-moderate MR is often associated with poor LV function, 'functional' in nature and associated with normal valves.

Tricuspid regurgitation (TR)

- Severity graded from 1 to 4, as for aortic and mitral regurgitation.

- Mild TR is detectable in most normal people.

- More severe TR is common in severe biventricular failure, mitral stenosis, cor pulmonale and any other cause of pulmonary hypertension.

- The peak systolic pressure gradient across the tricuspid valve (peak systolic TVG) can be calculated from the peak TR velocity. In the absence of pulmonary stenosis: peak pulmonary artery pressure = peak systolic TVG + right atrial pressure

- This is often simplified to: peak pulmonary artery pressure = peak systolic TVG + 10 mmHg. Note: in the presence of a very high JVP or CVP, right atrial pressure is significantly > 10 mmHg and pulmonary pressures may be significantly underestimated.

Further reading

Daniel WG, Mügge A. Transesophageal echocardiography. *N Engl J Med* 1995; **332**: 1268–79.

Feigenbaum H. *Echocardiography*, 5th edn, 1994. Philadelphia: Lea & Febiger.

Rimington H, Chambers J. *Echocardiography. A Practical Guide for Reporting.* Parthenon, 1998. Carnforth, UK

References

1. Køber L, Torp-Pedersen C, Carlsen J *et al.* An echocardiographic method for selecting high risk patients shortly after acute myocardial infarction, for inclusion in multi-centre studies (as used in the TRACE study). *Eur Heart J* 1994; **15**: 1616–20.

2. Al-Khadra AS, Salem DN, Rand WM *et al.* Warfarin anticoagulation and survival: a cohort analysis from the studies of left ventricular dysfunction. *J Am Coll Cardiol* 1998; **31**: 749–53.

3. Ciaccheri M, Castelli G, Cecchi F *et al.* Lack of correlation between intracavity thrombosis detected by cross-sectional echocardiography and systemic emboli in patients with dilated cardiomyopathy. *Br Heart J* 1989; **62**: 26–9.

4. Wheeldon NM. Atrial fibrillation and anticoagulant therapy. *Eur Heart J* 1995; **16**: 302–12.

5. Zabalgoitia M, Halperin JL, Pearce LA *et al.* Transesophageal echocardiographic correlates of clinical risk of thromboembolism in nonvalvular atrial fibrillation. Stroke Prevention in Atrial Fibrillation III Investigators. *J Am Coll Cardiol* 1998; **31**: 1622–6.

6. Chirillo F, Totis O, Cavarzerani A *et al.* Usefulness of transthoracic and transesophageal echocardiography in recognition and management of cardiovascular injuries after blunt chest trauma. *Heart* 1996; **75**: 301–6.

9

MECHANICAL AIDS

Technological advances have produced mechanical aids that provide inotropic or chronotropic support either temporarily or permanently for diseased hearts. The aim is to discuss the role of such devices in the modern management of cardiac patients.

INTRA-AORTIC BALLOON COUNTERPULSATION (IABP)

IABP is a device that can provide temporary mechanical support to the circulation. Such devices often support the circulation while the myocardium recovers following cardiac surgery and can aid patients with cardiac disease that is amenable to surgical correction (including transplantation). It consists of an inflatable balloon attached to an external console. The balloon, which is usually 40–50 ml, is inserted either percutaneously via the femoral artery or by surgical 'cut down' and is positioned just distal to the origin of the left subclavian artery.

It is triggered to inflate with helium or carbon dioxide immediately after aortic valve closure, and deflates as the aortic valve opens in early systole. Timing is usually linked to the ECG R-wave and can be checked by reference to the aortic pressure trace. Inflation should occur at the dicrotic notch and an augmented diastolic wave should be apparent.

The net effect is an increase in coronary blood flow, cardiac output, aortic diastolic and mean pressures, and a reduction in LV end-diastolic pressure and systemic vascular resistance (after load reduction). The IABP is unique in that it can improve cardiac output without increasing myocardial oxygen demand.

While full support is required, all or every second heart beat is supported. As the patient improves weaning is usually achieved by decreasing the ratio of supported beats, e.g. to 1:3 and then 1:4 before removal. Alternatively some prefer to reduce the balloon volume gradually.

Problems related to poor timing of inflation include:

- If inflation is too soon – increase in afterload as inflates during systole obstructing LV outflow.

- If inflation is too late – reduced beneficial effect

- If deflation is too early – reduced beneficial effect.

- If deflation too late – increase in afterload as still inflated at start of systole.

Indications

- Refractory ventricular failure.

- Cardiogenic shock.

- Refractory unstable angina.

- Impending myocardial infarction with hypotension.

- Mechanical complications due to acute myocardial infarction: ventricular septal defect, mitral regurgitation, and papillary muscle rupture.

- Cardiac support for high-risk general surgery.

- Weaning from cardiopulmonary bypass.

- Support and stabilization during or after coronary angiography and angioplasty.

Contraindications

- Severe aortic regurgitation.

- Abdominal or aortic aneurysm.

- Severe peripheral vascular disease.

Advantages

- Increase in cardiac output by 20–40% (due to a decrease in myocardial oxygen consumption from a reduction in LV filling pressure, and an increase in coronary blood flow augmented coronary perfusion pressure).

- Easily placed in > 90% of patients.

- Prolonged treatment is possible.

- Requires only a moderate-sized sheath (8.0–10.5 F) compared with other support devices or sheathless insertion can be done.

Disadvantages

- High incidence (9–43%) of vascular complications, including AV fistula, pseudo-aneurysm, ileofemoral thrombosis and local bleeding.

- Requires stable cardiac rhythm for effective diastolic augmentation.

- Moderate haemolysis and thrombocytopenia are common (although platelet counts < 50000 are unusual).

TEMPORARY CARDIAC PACING

Familiarity with temporary cardiac pacing is important for those involved in permanent cardiac pacing and for those involved with treatment of patients in intensive care units, coronary care units and post-surgical wards. The knowledge of indications, techniques and routes of implantation is required for safe and reliable pacing.

Indications

Third-degree AV block:

- Symptomatic congenital complete heart block

- Symptomatic acquired complete heart block

- Postoperative symptomatic complete block

- Symptomatic 2nd degree AV block.

- Acute myocardial infarction:

- Symptomatic bradycardia complicated by cardiac decompensation

Complete heart block

- General anaesthesia – patients with second- or third-degree AV block should have a temporary pacemaker preoperatively.

- Tachycardia – prevention or treatment:

- Bradycardia-dependent arrhythmias

- Long QT syndrome with ventricular arrhythmias

- Termination of atrial flutter or ventricular tachycardia

Temporary pacemaker placement

- Temporary pacing is usually performed by a transvenous approach. The clinical need determines the urgency with which pacing is required and therefore often the venous access chosen.

- Either external, transcutaneous or oesophageal approaches are possible, short-term alternatives in emergencies to stabilize a patient.

Transvenous pacing

Temporary transvenous ventricular pacing is usually carried out by placing a transvenous bipolar pacing electrode. Access to the venous system is possible from several sites including the subclavian, external and internal jugular, brachial and femoral veins. Selection of specific approach depends on clinical conditions and the experience of the operator. Insertion should be done under sterile aseptic conditions.

Femoral venous puncture is particularly useful in a cardiac arrest situation but should be reserved for short-term emergency purposes due to electrode instability and risk of venous thrombosis and infection.

The placement of a temporary ventricular pacing lead is usually achieved with the aid of fluoroscopic guidance with the tip of the electrode positioned at the right ventricular apex. In many patients a loop is fashioned within the right atrium, rotated counter-clockwise across the tricuspid valve. Crossing of the tricuspid valve is usually associated with the provocation of ventricular ectopic beats. If these are not provoked, then it may be the coronary sinus has been entered. A lateral screen view will show that the electrode is pointing posteriorly. The electrode in the right ventricular apex points anteriorly.

It is possible to place an electrode catheter without X-ray screening particularly if one is chosen with a balloon tip. Balloon flotation catheters do not require fluoroscopy and its insertion is similar to a pulmonary artery catheter. Intracardiac electrograms can help position the leads. However, balloon flotation catheters may not maintain stable pacing positions.

Pacing

When a stable electrode position is achieved, the pacing threshold should be ascertained. This is the minimal voltage necessary for a pacing stimulus to capture the ventricles consistently. This should be < 1 volt although, in an emergency, a less than optimal pacing threshold may have to be accepted. In a conscious patient, the stability of the pacing lead should be testing ensuring consisting pacing during deep inspiration, coughing or sniffing. To ensure lead stability, the electrode should be securely sutured to the skin at point of entry.

Atrial lead placement

Ventricular pacing does result in atrioventricular dissociation and hence a reduction in cardiac output. Both atria and ventricles can be paced sequentially producing important benefits in cardiac function.

A temporary atrial lead is placed in the right atrial appendage, which allows for stable reliable pacing. The currently available temporary leads have a preshaped 'J' that facilitates right atrial appendage positioning. This is obviously easier from either the jugular or subclavian approach. Right atrial position is characterized by a typical medial and lateral movement during atrial systole.

An alternative to separate ventricular and atrial leads are a 'single-pass' multipolar catheter with electrodes placed against the right ventricle and the lateral border of the right atrium. There are also pulmonary artery catheters with atrial and ventricular pacing ports.

Epicardial pacing

Epicardial temporary pacing is used exclusively in patients undergoing cardiac surgery. These are sometimes placed prophylactically in all patients undergoing cardiac surgery but often only in patients in whom AV block develops during the procedure or pacing is required to wean patients from cardiopulmonary bypass.

Electrodes used are stainless steel Teflon-coated wires sutured loosely on to the epicardium brought out through the chest wall.

Oesophageal pacing

The oesophagus can be used for obtaining cardiac electrograms and for cardiac pacing. A coronary sinus lead can be placed into the oesophagus and the catheter advanced into position to record the largest and most distinct atrial electrogram. It can be used for overdrive pacing, particularly for atrial flutter. Also will demonstrate AV dissociation in VT to aid diagnosis if the diagnosis is in doubt.

A long impulse duration is necessary (10 ms) to avoid patient discomfort.

External transcutaneous pacing

External cardiac pacing devices are designed for easy and rapid use in emergency situations. It is particularly useful to support symptomatic bradyarrhythmia until a transvenous pacemaker can be placed but can be uncomfortable for a conscious, alert, patient.

Complications

Complications can be associated with the venous access site as for central venous catheters (see Chapter 5) and is lower via the internal jugular venous route.

- The most common complication with temporary pacing is lead dislodgement. If there is evidence of failure to pace and/or sense, repositioning of the electrode may be required.

- Perforation of the right ventricle is a recognized complication and may become evident clinically because of a friction rub, loss of pacing, diaphragmatic stimulation or rarely by pericardial tamponade.

- It is important to pay particular attention to a scrupulous aseptic technique and care of the access site. Local skin infection is particularly common if the lead is in position for any length of time. If the temporary pacing lead is left in position for prolonged periods, then bacteraemia may result usually due to a skin organism. It is particularly important that the sheath used for venous access is pulled back when the lead is in place so as not to produce a portal for bacterial organisms.

- Severe sepsis and septic shock should be treated in the usual manner with blood cultures, swabs, appropriate antibiotics and removal of the infected lead (see Chapter 7).

- Any intracardiac catheter can produce arrhythmias, the most common of which are ventricular ectopics and occasionally ventricular tachycardia. This can be particularly a problem if the pacing failed to sense a native QRS complex with resultant pacing stimulus delivered during repolarization (T-wave). Ventricular tachycardia or ventricular fibrillation may rarely be induced.

PERMANENT PACEMAKERS

Permanent pacemakers are based on the same principles, but the pulse generator is implanted subcutaneously in a pre-pectoral pocket. The electrodes are placed in the RV for ventricular pacing and right atrial appendage for atrial pacing.

Indications

This includes conditions in which implantations of a permanent cardiac pacemaker are thought necessary provided that the conditions are chronic and recurrent and not due to any transient cause such as acute myocardial ischaemia (MI), electrolyte imbalance and drug interactions. They are based on AHA/ACC guidelines (see further reading).

Group 1 indications – pacemaker mandatory:

- Acquired complete AV block.

- Congenital complete AV block with severe bradycardia or significant physiological deficit.

- Symptomatic Mobitz 2 AV block.

- Symptomatic Mobitz 1 secondary degree AV block with symptoms related to haemodynamic instability.

- Symptomatic sinus bradycardia (syncope, congestive cardiac failure).

- Symptomatic sinus bradycardia that is the consequence of long-term required drug treatment.

- Sinus node dysfunction and symptomatic bradycardia with or without tachycardia. This includes the tachycardia/bradycardia syndrome, sino-atrial block and sinus arrest.

- Sinus node dysfunction with or without symptoms when there are potentially life-threatening arrhythmias secondary to bradycardia.

- Carotid sinus hypersensitivity. This is an indication in patients who suffer from near syncope or syncope with evidence of sinus node dysfunction on a tilt table test or carotid sinus massage, pauses, sinus arrest or complete AV block for at least 3 s.

Group 2 indications include conditions in which the use of a cardiac pacemaker may be found acceptable and necessary, and there is evidence that pacemaker implantation will assist overall management:

- Congenital complete heart block with less severe bradycardia.

- Bi- or tri-fascicular block accompanied by a syncope attributed to transient complete heart block and other causes of syncope have been excluded.

- Prophylactic pacemaker use after recovery from an acute MI during which there is transient, complete or Mobitz 2 second-degree AV block.

- Asymptomatic Mobitz 2 second-degree AV block.

- Symptomatic sinus bradycardia (heart rate < 45 beats/min) that is a consequence of long-term necessary drug treatment for which there is no acceptable alternative.

- Overdrive pacing in patients with recurrent and refractory ventricular tachycardia to prevent ventricular tachycardia.

- Dual-chamber pacing with short AV delay reducing symptoms of LV outflow tract obstructure in some patients with hypertrophic cardiomyopathy.

Group 3 includes conditions that are considered unsupported by adequate evidence to benefit from permanent pacing and should not be considered appropriate uses of pacemakers in the absence of indications in groups 1 and 2:

- Syncope of undetermined cause – syncope requires extensive investigation including neurological evaluation.

- Sinus bradycardia without significant symptoms.

- Sino-atrial disease without significant symptoms.

- Prolonged RR intervals with atrial fibrillation without symptoms.

- Bradycardia during sleep.

- Right bundle branch block with left axis deviation without syncope or other symptoms of AV block.

- Asymptomatic second-degree Mobitz 1 (Wenckebach) AV block.

- First-degree AV block.

Pacemaker indications are changing all the time. Newer indications include:

- Biventricular pacing for heart failure – recent studies have revealed improvement in haemodynamic symptoms in patients with heart failure and intraventricular conduction delays. Intraventricular conduction delay results in abnormal electrical depolarization with mechanical asynchrony of the ventricles. Resynchronization using biventricular pacing with leads in the right ventricular apex and a second lead placed in a vein in the posterolateral wall of the heart via the coronary sinus may be beneficial. This technique may also play a role to stabilize patients before definitive cardiac surgery or cardiac transplantation.

- Multisite atrial pacing to prevent atrial fibrillation. There have been studies performed with bi-atrial pacing with atrial leads in the right atrial appendage and either atrial septum or at a site near the orifice of the coronary sinus to reduce interatrial conduction delay. This may have a role in the prevention of atrial fibrillation in paroxysmal atrial fibrillation or post-cardiac surgery.

System construction

The pacing system consists of a generator and one or two pacing leads. The pulse generator has three basic components:

A battery (power source), timer and an electrical impulse performer. The generator is hermetically sealed and the circuitry and battery are housed within a titanium canister attached to the header block containing the electrode connections. The leads are insulated, non-thrombogenic, biocompatible with good conductivity. The conducting wire is of metal alloy covered with an insulating layer of silicon or polyurethane.

The uninsulated distal end of the lead is attached to the myocardium using either passive or active fixation. Passive fixation involves the anchoring system of Tines, which are entangled in the RV trabeculae or the pectinate muscles of the right atrial appendage. Active fixation involves penetration of the muscle with a screw mechanism. This is particularly useful in patients with significant tricuspid regurgitation, in whom passive fixation has failed, or patient's post-cardiac-surgery.

Modern permanent pacemakers are all multi-programmable and have the capacity to sense intrinsic electrical activity and are therefore programmed to respond to a sensed cardiac event by not pacing for a preset interval. Modern developments have led to a physiological approach to cardiac pacing with dual-chamber pacing becoming increasingly more common (at least 60% of all implants). Dual-chamber pacing offers superior haemodynamics leading to better effort tolerance, a lower prevalence of atrial arrhythmias and the ability to prevent 'pacemaker syndrome' (a fall in blood pressure and dizziness precipitated by ventricular pacing). The international code for pacing is given in table 1.

Newer pacing facilities include automatic mode switching for patients prone to paroxysmal atrial arrhythmias. The pacemaker will function as a normal dual chamber pacemaker (DDD) while the patient is in sinus rhythm but will switch to either DDI or VVI at the onset of atrial arrhythmias so as not to track fast atrial fibrillation or other atrial arrhythmias.[1]

Complications

Complications are often related to the implant as per temporary pacing. Other complications are:

- Electromyographic interference (usually confined to unipolar pacing systems). Myopotentials generated from underlying muscle can be sensed by the pacemaker as spontaneous cardiac activity with inappropriate inhibition of pacing activity. This can be overcome by alterations in sensitivity or polarity.

- Pacing lead complications can include exit block due to excessive fibrous tissue formation around the tip of the pacing lead. This is most likely to occur within the first 3 weeks to 3 months after implantation. Modern leads have a low surface area, porous surface electrodes and steroid elusion, which rarely gives rise to this complication.

- Lead fracture usually at the point where the lead enters the venous system, at the site of fixation suture or at sites of excessive angulation can lead to this relatively rare complication. This can be detected radiographically.

- Insulation breakdown allows leakage of current that may cause stimulation of adjacent muscles and premature battery depletion.

Table 1 NASPE/BPEG* Generic (NBG) pacemaker code

Position Category	I Chamber(s) paced	II Chamber(s) sensed	III Response to sensing	IV Programmability, rate modulation, etc.	V Anti-tachyarrhythmia function(s)
	O = None	O = None	O = None	O = None	O = None
	A = Atrium	A = Atrium	T = Triggered	P = Simple programmable	P = Pacing (anti-tachyarrhythmia)
	V = Ventricle	V = Ventricle	I = Inhibited	M = Multi-programmable	S = Shock
	D = Dual (A + V)	D = Dual (A + V)	D = Dual (T + I)	C = Communicating	D = Dual (P + S)
				R = Rate modulation	

*NASPE = North American Society of Pacing and Electrophysiology; BPEG = British Pacing and Electrophysiology Group
See Reference 3.

- Premature battery depletion and failure is an occasional complication.

- Diaphragmatic stimulation can at times occur. This can sometimes be overcome by reducing the output of the generator but occasionally lead repositioning is required.

Pacemaker interference – practical considerations

Interference of pacemaker function can occur and the following points should be considered:

Cardioversion or defibrillation

- Defibrillation pads should optimally be placed antero-posteriorly so minimizing the chance of placing a paddle over a pulse generator or having the current path go directly to the lead system. The pad should be at least 10–15 cm away from the pacemaker itself.

- The pacemaker should be interrogated following the procedure to ensure that the pacing function has not been changed.

Electrocautery/diathermy

- The most common problem encountered with this form of treatment is pacemaker inhibition. If the electrical intervention is brief, this is not a concern.

- Ideally bipolar diathermy should be used.

- The electrode should be at least 15 cm away from the pacemaker.

- Consideration should be given to reprogramming the pacemaker to an asynchronous mode to avoid intermittent inhibition (VOO or fixed rate). This is particularly important in patients who are pacemaker-dependent.

- In an emergency, a magnet can convert the pacemaker to a fixed rate mode, thus avoiding inhibition.

- The pacemaker should be re-interrogated after diathermy is finished to ensure it is in the correct mode.

Magnetic resonance imaging (MRI)

- MRI can affect normal pacemaker and operation. At the very least exposure to MRI causes all pacemakers to revert to an asynchronous mode (VOO). Theoretically, due to the sometimes short radio-frequency pulse periods, patients with susceptible pacemakers could theoretically be paced with rates as high as 3000 beats/min.

- In general, therefore, MRI should be avoided in patients with implanted pacemakers.

- If the pacemaker can be programmed to OOO mode (off), a non-pace-maker-dependent patient can be scanned safely.

- There have been cases where MRI scanning is vital and pacemakers have been explanted temporarily in the non-dependent patient. However, there is obviously a risk of infection with this approach.

Lithotripsy

- Extracorporeal shock wave lithotripsy used for the treatment of nephrolithiasis or cholelithiasis potentially can interfere with permanent pacemaker function. Lithotripsy does not interfere with a fixed rate VVI pacing as long as the focal point of the lithotripter is at least 15 cm from the pacemaker.

- In patients with dual-chamber pacing, synchronization of the lithotripter with the atrial output can result in inhibition of ventricular output. Therefore, the pacemaker should be programmed to VVI or VOO mode (fixed rate) for the duration of the treatment.

Transcutaneous nerve stimulation (TENS)

- This form of treatment appears safe in most patients with permanent pacing and rarely causes inhibition, interference or reprogramming.

- It is best to avoid applying the stimulator to a vector or path that would be parallel to the pacing lead.

- Pacemaker-dependent patients should be monitored during the TENS treatment to be certain of no inhibition.

Therapeutic radiation

- Diagnostic X-ray does not interfere with pacemaker function.

- Therapeutic radiation levels can damage pacemaker function and may be of sufficient intensity to result in complete failure or random damage to circuit components.

- In patients in whom the pacemaker is within the field of radiation such as carcinoma of the breast, the pulse generator should be moved to another site. If it is not in the field of radiation, it should be shielded to prevent damage.

Electroconvulsive therapy (ECT)

- ECT for treatment for depression does not usually result in pacemaker malfunction, but the pacemaker should be interrogated following ECT to ensure that it is still programmed correctly.

Implantable cardiac defibrillator (ICD)[2]

Sudden cardiac death, secondary to ventricular arrhythmias, is a common cause of mortality. Cardioversion/defibrillation is important in the management of these arrhythmias. The development of the ICD is a major advance and with increasing numbers used it is important to be aware of their mechanism of operation. Older ICD used to have pulse generators weighing > 200 g. These generators were implanted in the abdominal position in the anterior or posterior rectus sheath. Newer, much smaller generators are now implanted in the pectoral position either subpectorally or subcutaneously as with permanent pacemakers.

- Up until 1990 all devices used epicardial patches requiring a thoracotomy. Now virtually all devices consist of a ventricular transvenous lead.

Indications

General indications include:

- One or more episodes of spontaneous sustained VT or VF in a patient in whom electrophysiological (EP) testing and/or spontaneous arrhythmias cannot be used accurately to predict efficacy of therapy.

- Recurrent spontaneous sustained VT and/or VF despite anti-arrhythmic therapy or where the use of drugs is limited by side-effects or intolerance.

- Persistent inducibility of clinically relevant sustained VT or VF at EP study despite drug therapy in a patient with spontaneous sustained VT or VF.

ICD implantation is not recommended in patients in whom ventricular arrhythmias occur in the setting of acute myocardial ischaemia or infarction, or reversible toxicological and metabolic abnormalities.

Patients successfully resuscitated following cardiac arrest are at high risk of sudden cardiac death, recurrence (up to 50% within 12 months). Those with poor LV function and ventricular arrhythmias have an increased risk of subsequent cardiac arrest. Recent trial data have extended the indications to include patients with poor LV function and non-sustained VT on Holter monitoring.

Implantation

Implants are now carried out under local anaesthetic with IV sedation. A RV lead is positioned passively in the RV apex or actively at other sites in the RV with either a single defibrillation coil within the RV or a second coil on the same lead in the supra vena cava. The device will 'shock' between the generator and the defibrillation coil on the electrode.

In most patients this will result in adequate defibrillation thresholds (DFT), but some patients will also need the placement of a subcutaneous patch or electrode array.

These single-chamber devices are the most commonly implanted ICD. However, with improvements in technology, the dual-chamber devices are now also implanted with an additional bipolar atrial sensing electrode, which can result in dual-chamber pacing and better discrimination between atrial and ventricular arrhythmias.

ICD function

Most devices will allow several levels of detection and therapy. This 'tiered therapy' can allow for differing treatments for slow VT, fast VT and ventricular fibrillation. The therapies can consist of anti-tachycardia pacing (ATP), cardioversion shocks and defibrillation shocks.

- Anti-tachycardia pacing can be an effective treatment to terminate VT with using either programmed extra-stimuli, a delivery of a train of stimuli and fixed coupling interval (burst pacing) or delivery of a burst of extra-stimuli where the coupling interval becomes progressively shorter (ramp pacing).

- VT can be terminated by low energy synchronized shock (cardioversion).

- For the treatment of fast VT and VF, defibrillation up to 35 joules can be delivered from the devices.

- ICD also function as a Holter monitor with the capture of an episode showing surface and intracardiac electrograms.

Atrial defibrillators[3]

Atrial defibrillators have been developed for patients either with atrial fibrillation in association with serious ventricular arrhythmias or primarily as the treatment for atrial fibrillation. These devices can be automatic or, more commonly, patient- or physician-activated for termination of fast atrial fibrillation in patients with paroxysmal atrial fibrillation. The numbers of these implants are still relatively low in the UK.

Temporary internal atrial cardioversion

There are devices available for internal transvenous atrial cardioversion. Internal cardioversion has the advantage of lower energies (0.5–15 joules) delivered directly to the atria.[4] There are data available indicating a much better success rate for internal versus external cardioversion.

The catheter is floated into the pulmonary (preferably left) artery. The distal electrode array is positioned in the pulmonary artery in a proximal electrode array in the right atrium. Atrial cardioversion is performed with R-wave synchronization. There is also the facility to pace to terminate atrial tachyarrhythmias with atrial and ventricular tachycardia pacing and sensing and haemodynamic monitoring.

The advantages of this form of treatment is that it requires only mild sedation and eliminates the trauma and discomfort associated with high-energy external cardioversion. This procedure has also been successful in patients who have failed previous external cardioversions.

Miscellaneous devices

There have been a number of devices used temporarily to support either LV or RV function in patients who cannot be sustained by pharmacological therapy and/or intra-aortic balloon assistance. For patients in whom recovery of LV function is anticipated or as a bridge to cardiac transplantation, several LV assist devices have been developed consisting of a pump with afferent and efferent conduits attached to the LV apex and ascending thoracic aorta respectively.

A number of permanent LV assist devices and totally artificial hearts are also currently in development and/or testing and are therefore not widely available outside of major cardiac transplant units.

Further reading

ACC/AHA Guidelines for Implantation of Cardiac Pacemakers and Antiarrhythmia Devices: A Report of the American College of Cardiology/ American Heart Association Task Force of Practice Guidelines (Committee on Pacemaker Implantation). *J Am Coll Cardiol* 1998: **31**; 1175–209.

Bernstein AD, Camm AJ, Fletcher RD *et al.* The NASPE/BPEG generic pacemaker code for antibradyarrhythmia and adaptive-rate pacing and antitachyarrhythmia devices. *PACE* 1987: **10**; 794–9.

Clarke M, Sutton R, Ward D *et al.* Recommendations for pacemaker prescription for symptomatic bradycardia. Report of a working party of the BPEG. *Br Heart J* 1991: **66**; 185–91.

Connolly SJ. Implantable cardioverter defibrillators – for whom? *Lancet*; **352**: 338–40. 1998

Underwood MJ, Firmin RK, Graham TR. Current concepts in the use of intra-aortic balloon counterpulsation. *Br J Hosp Med* 1993: **50**; 391–7.

References

1. Attuel P, Pelleris D, Mugica J *et al.* DDD pacing: an effective treatment modality for recurrent atrial arrhythmias. *PACE* 1988: **11**; 1647–54.

2. Moss AJ, Hall WJ, Cannom DS *et al.* Improved survival with an implanted defibrillator in patients with coronary disease at high risk for ventricular arrhythmia. *N Engl J Med* 1996; **335**; 1933–40.

3. Saksena S, Prakash A, Mangeon L *et al.* Clinical efficacy and safety of atrial defibrillator using biphasic shocks and current nonthoracotomy endocardial lead configurations. *Am J Cardiol* 1995; **76**: 913–21.

4. Santini M, Pandozi C, Toscano S *et al.* Low energy intracardiac cardioversion of persistent atrial fibrillation. *PACE* 1998: **21**; 2641–50.

10

CATHETER-BASED TREATMENTS FOR ACUTE CARDIAC EMERGENCIES

Since the initial application of balloon angioplasty to the treatment of coronary artery disease, there has been an explosive growth in the field of interventional cardiology. A variety of new devices, in addition to adjunctive pharmacological therapies, have been developed to treat lesions in patients with high-risk characteristics. Also, catheter-based techniques have been developed to treat acute presentations of a number of other cardiac conditions in adults and children. Interventional catheter-based treatments in paediatric cardiology, however, have not been discussed here.

EMERGENCY CORONARY ANGIOPLASTY

In the setting of acute ischaemic syndromes, percutaneous transluminal coronary angioplasty (PTCA) can be used to:

- restore flow in an acutely occluded coronary artery during acute myocardial infarction (MI) – primary or direct angioplasty;

- restore patency after failed thrombolysis – rescue angioplasty;

- treat recurrent ischaemia following acute MI; and

- prevent recurrent ischaemia in patients with unstable angina.

Technique

When performing PTCA, arterial access is obtained via the femoral, brachial or radial artery. A guiding catheter is fed retrograde to the aorta and placed at the coronary ostium. Angiography is then performed to delineate the coronary anatomy and areas of stenoses or occlusion. Coronary flow at angiography is graded according to the TIMI (thrombolysis in MI) classification:

- TIMI grade 0 = no flow.
- TIMI grade 1 = minimal dye penetration.
- TIMI grade 2 = partial, subnormal flow.
- TIMI grade 3 = normal flow.

Coronary angiographic assessment provides a powerful means of preprocedural risk stratification for PTCA. A number of angiographic risk factors that have been identified for a coronary lesion. The American College of Cardiology and the American Heart Association have incorporated these risk factors into a scheme that classifies lesions as type A, B and C according to expected procedural success rates and risks of complications.

- Type A lesions – associated with high (> 85%) procedural success rate and low risk of complications have one or more of the following characteristics: discrete (< 10 mm length), concentric, little or no calcification, readily accessible, non-angulated segment, smooth contour, less than totally occlusive, not ostial in location, no major branch involvement, absence of thrombus.

- Type B lesions – associated with moderate success (60–85%) and moderate risk of complication have one or more of the following characteristics: tubular (10–20 mm), eccentric, moderate tortuosity of proximal segment, moderately angulated segment, irregular contour, moderate-to-heavy calcification, total occlusion < 3 months old, ostial in location, bifurcation lesions requiring double guidewires, some thrombus present.

- Type C lesions – associated with low success rate (< 60%) and high risk of complications have one or more of the following features: diffuse (> 2 cm length), excessive tortuosity of proximal segment, extremely angulated segments, total occlusion > 3 months old, inability to protect major sidebranches, degenerated vein grafts with friable lesions.

A suitably identified lesion is crossed with a guidewire. A balloon, appropriately sized using quantitative coronary angiography, is then directed across the area of stenosis and inflated to nominal pressure for the size of the balloon or until the balloon is fully distended on fluoroscopy. In doing this, the area of atherosclerotic plaque is fractured and pushed into the wall of the coronary artery, thus reducing the area of original stenosis. During the procedure, heparin is used to prevent thrombogenesis and often intracoronary nitrate is used to stimulate intracoronary vasodilatation. Post-dilation angiography is performed to define any residual stenosis.

No reflow phenomenon

This refers to the failure to achieve reperfusion after a prolonged period of ischaemia. It is caused largely by microvascular damage. It is contained within areas of myocardium already necrotic at the time of onset of reperfusion. It may be secondary to distal embolization of clot or atherosclerotic plaque.

Limitations to angioplasty

- Difficult arterial access (e.g. severe peripheral arterial disease).

- Inability to receive aspirin (relative contraindication) or heparin (i.e. previous heparin-induced thrombocytopenia).

- Left main stem coronary stenosis with no functioning bypass graft available (relative contraindication) or stenosis in last remaining patent coronary artery.

- Inability to reach or cross infarct-related occlusion.

PRIMARY ANGIOPLASTY

- Definition – coronary angioplasty performed **without prior** thrombolytic therapy during acute MI.

Requirements for primary PTCA

- Evidence of acute MI.

- Access to catheterization laboratory with experienced cardiologist.

- Ability to perform PTCA within 90 min of presentation.

- Patients with contraindications to thrombolytics or cardiogenic shock.

Advantages of primary PTCA over thrombolysis

- Excellent reperfusion rates – primary PTCA can achieve more rapid and complete reperfusion, as evidenced by 90-min TIMI grade 3 flow rates of about 90%, as compared with the best normal flow rate reported with conventional thrombolytic agents (accelerated tissue plasminogen activator) of 65%.

- Less residual stenosis – may contribute to more rapid recovery of left ventricular function after reperfusion. Re-occlusion rates are also lower. Striking results have been obtained with primary angioplasty in selected centres. There have been a number of randomized trials of primary angioplasty versus thrombolytic therapy.[1-4] The benefit of primary PTCA was particularly marked in higher risk patients, who were older or had anterior infarctions.

- Prompt identification of reperfusion.

- Identification of severity and extent of coronary artery disease facilitating triage and enhancing the therapeutic decision process.

- Effective for patients with haemodynamic instability.

- Facilitates access for placement of haemodynamic support devices, e.g. intra-aortic balloon pump.

Disadvantages

- Requires prompt, easy access to catheterization laboratory.

- Costs of maintenance of 24-h laboratory facilities.

- Needs operator experience.

- Mortality among the minority of patients with failed primary angioplasty is excessively high in the range of 25–40%. Potential explanations for this finding include haemodynamic disturbances during the procedure and distal embolization.

The facilities for performing primary angioplasty are not present in the majority of hospitals treating patients with MI and the cost and logistics of providing universal availability of primary angioplasty is prohibitive.

RESCUE ANGIOPLASTY

- Definition – use of PTCA in patients in whom reperfusion has not occurred after thrombolysis as opposed to 'immediate' angioplasty, where PTCA is done after thrombolysis whether reperfusion has occurred or not.

Inclusion criteria for rescue PTCA

- Evidence of MI with:

- persistent chest pain after thrombolysis and/or

- persistent ST-elevation after thrombolysis

- Haemodynamic instability (cardiogenic shock).

Results from randomized trials of rescue PTCA have shown that rescue PTCA might help in failed thrombolysis but fall short of proving benefit.[5] The strategy itself has limitations – the problem being that by the time patients have presented and received thrombolysis and failed reperfusion has become apparent, the infarct is well established and the microvascular damage is extensive. Rescue angioplasty is more likely to be accompanied by no reflow. If angioplasty is undertaken, adjunctive treatments such as abcixmab or intra-aortic balloon pumping may be required.

Identification of better means rapidly to assess reperfusion status as well as improved antithrombotic regimens should further improve the results of therapy in patients with failed reperfusion.

PTCA for treatment of cardiogenic shock (see Chapter 13)

The development of cardiogenic shock in association with acute MI identifies a patient with an extremely poor prognosis. Even in the best of circumstances mortality rate from cardiogenic shock in thrombolytic patients remains very high. Similar to the treatment of acute MI without shock, the most essential aspect of therapy in acute infarction with cardiogenic shock is achieving infarct artery patency. The SHOCK (should we emergently revascularize occluded coronaries for cardiogenic shock) trial evaluated early revascularization, either primary angioplasty or bypass surgery, in patients with cardiogenic shock.[6] In this trial, emergency revascularization (i.e. procedure performed for < 12 h after the diagnosis of shock) did not significantly reduce overall mortality rate at 30 days, but at 6 months there was a significant survival benefit.

Immediate PTCA

The combination of inevitable procedural delay associated with primary PTCA and the promising results of IV thrombolytic therapy led to the anticipation that follow on PTCA immediately after thrombolytic therapy would improve the initial advantage of thrombolytic reperfusion. However, trial evidence supports the view that in clinically stable patients following successful pharmacological coronary recanalization nothing is to be gained by immediate PTCA.[7] Possible explanations for this include exacerbation of platelet activation and thrombosis at the site of plaque rupture and increased bleeding including haemorrhagic dissections of the target vessel.

PTCA in unstable angina

Successful PTCA in unstable angina results in symptomatic improvement as well as both regional and global improvement of ischaemic left ventricular dysfunction.

Acute complications of PTCA are slightly higher in patients with unstable as opposed to stable angina. The late outcomes are similar.[8]

Risk factors for a procedure-related complication include:

- Very severe degree of stenosis.

- Presence of thrombus.

- ST-segment elevations or persistent T-wave inversions

- Number of lesions attempted.

The incidence of ischaemic complications in patients with unstable angina undergoing PTCA is reduced by treatment with the monoclonal anti-IIb/IIIa antibody 7E3 (see below on adjunctive pharmacotherapy).[9]

Complications of PTCA

- Acute vessel closure.

- Death.

- Restenosis.

- Emergency coronary artery bypass grafting (about 1.4%).

- Cardiac arrhythmias – more often with right coronary artery.

- Haemorrhage requiring blood transfusion.

Acute vessel closure

Abrupt vessel occlusion is the major cause of death and MI after balloon angioplasty. Acute closure is associated with a 25–30% incidence of Q-wave MI and even higher rates of non-Q-wave MI. The incidence of abrupt vessel occlusion after angioplasty ranges from 4 to 10%.

The mechanisms of abrupt vessel occlusion include extensive medial dissection with a dissecting haematoma that is under pressure and compresses the true lumen, intraluminal thrombus, immediate elastic recoil, vasoconstriction, or prolapse of flap or plaque into lumen.

Correlates of mortality after abrupt closure

- Female gender.

- Age > 65–70 years.

- History of congestive heart failure.

- LV ejection fraction < 30%.

- Unstable angina.

- Multivessel or left main coronary disease.

- Collaterals arising from the target vessel.

- Proximal right coronary artery dilatation.

- New onset angina.

Restenosis

The principal factor limiting long-term benefit of coronary angioplasty is restenosis, the angiographic renarrowing of the vessel lumen following successful balloon dilatation of a vascular lesion. Restenosis has traditionally been an angiographic diagnosis, defined as > 50% diameter stenosis at follow-up angiography. The most common manifestation of restenosis is recurrence of anginal chest pain. The pathogenesis of restenosis is complex and likely to be multi-factorial. The mechanism of restenosis differs significantly from *de novo* atherosclerosis and involves release of growth factors from activated platelets with subsequent invasion of the arterial wound by macrophages and modulation of smooth muscle cells to their proliferative phase leading to neo-intimal hyperplasia and restenosis.

Clinical, anatomical and procedural correlates of restenosis

Factors related to restenosis can conveniently and logically be grouped into three broad categories:

- Patient-related factors – unstable or variant angina, diabetes mellitus, male gender, smoking, hypercholesterolaemia, end-stage renal disease.

- Lesion-related factors – severe, bulky pre-angioplasty stenosis, proximal stenosis, left anterior descending artery stenosis, saphenous vein graft stenosis, chronic total occlusion, lesion calcification, bend stenosis, bifurcation stenosis, small vessels.

- Procedural-related factors – post-angioplasty residual stenosis > 30%; use of undersized balloon.

INTRACORONARY STENTS

Coronary stenting was developed as a counter to the two major limitations of PTCA: abrupt vessel closure and coronary restenosis. Since coronary stenting was first approved for elective implantation in 1994, the growth in use of the procedure has been explosive.

Technique

Stents are flexible endovascular prostheses. The stent is mounted on a balloon catheter and with the aid of fluoroscopic screening and radiopaque balloon markers is positioned across the stenotic lesion, which has usually been predilated with a balloon. Inflation of the balloon results in expansion and deployment of the stent circumferentially in apposition to the endothelial surface of the coronary artery.

Stents may be distinguished according to several factors:

- Type of delivery system – balloon mounted with expansion on balloon inflation, self expanding with expansion after retraction of a protective sheath.

- Structural design – tubular, single coil with a variable sine wave or helical design, wire-mesh structure.

- Metal composition – stainless steel, tantalum, platinum, cobalt-based alloy.

- Metal thickness

- Vascular wall surface coverage

- Stent coatings – heparin, phosphorylcholine.

Indications for stenting in acute coronary syndromes[10]

- Improvement of outcomes of PTCA – stenting increases minimal coronary luminal diameter at a lesion site to a greater degree than PTCA alone. Randomized, controlled trial data suggest that stents decrease both the rate of angiographic restenosis and the need for repeat revascularization compared with PTCA alone. Maximizing vessel lumen is the crucial mechanism in restenosis reduction. Despite a higher degree of vascular reaction after stent placement, the impact of this neo-intimal proliferation is counterbalanced to some extent by the important acute gain in luminal dimension. Furthermore, vascular remodelling, which has an important role in the restenosis process after PTCA, is abolished by stent implantation.

- To treat acute or threatened vessel closure – stenting in acute coronary syndromes may be reserved as 'bailout' devices for failed balloon angioplasty.[11] The mechanical properties of stents enable cardiologists to scaffold the vessel wall, tacking up dissections that are the main contributor to acute or threatened vessel closure after PTCA. The rate of emergency CABG has subsequently declined from 6% in the prestent era to < 0.5% in high-volume centres because of bailout stenting. However, it is not a foolproof safety net.

- To treat acute MI – data now exist to support that a primary stent strategy is safe and feasible in the majority of patients with an acute infarct undergoing mechanical reperfusion.[12,13] Several possible mechanisms may underlie the apparent safety of stenting in an obviously thrombotic environment. After primary PTCA for acute MI, the presence of dissection and a residual stenosis of > 30% have been shown to be major predictors of recurrent ischaemia and infarct-related artery re-occlusion. Both of these limitations of balloon dilatation are routinely overcome by stenting. Reinfarction after primary stenting may therefore be less common than after primary PTCA even if subacute thrombosis does rarely occur. Furthermore, the establishment by the stent of a wide lumen channel with brisk flow and no dissection planes may facilitate natural clot resolution by endogenous fibrinolysis.

Complications/limitations of coronary stenting in acute emergencies

- Inability or suboptimal stent deployment due to vessel tortuosity, diffuse disease, haemodynamic instability, extreme calcification of lesion.

- Difficult stent implantation procedure due to major dissection.

- Side branch occlusion due to inadvertent closure or sacrifice in favour of main branch.

- No reflow phenomenon during stent implantation-plaque embolization.

- Acute thrombotic occlusion.

Owing to the procedural limitations of angioplasty, apart from coronary stenting, there have been development of other devices and techniques of percutaneous revascularization such as coronary atherectomy, laser angioplasty and intracoronary radiation therapy combined with angioplasty, but their role and use in acute coronary syndromes has not yet been fully evaluated.

Adjunctive pharmacotherapy for coronary intervention

Coronary artery thrombosis plays a key role in acute coronary syndromes. Rupture of an atheromatous plaque exposes circulating platelets to ADP, thrombin and other thrombogenic material in the vessel wall, all of which results in platelet activation. This subsequently leads to expression of the glycoprotein IIb/IIIa receptor on the platelet surface, which then becomes capable of binding fibrinogen between adjacent platelets to form platelet aggregates. It is on the rich phospholipid surface of the platelet aggregate that coagulation with the generation of thrombin and the conversion of fibrinogen to fibrin occurs. Therefore, the development and usage of antiplatelet and antithrombin therapies has proved invaluable in reducing the likelihood of acute thrombotic complications following high-risk coronary interventions.[14]

Antiplatelet agents

Aspirin

Aspirin prevents platelet aggregation by irreversibly inhibiting the cyclo-oxygenase concerned with the formation of thromboxane A_2, one of several pathways through which platelets are activated. Aspirin therapy is recommended in all patients with acute coronary syndromes because it prevents recurrent ischaemic events and improves survival. Dosage: 75–150 mg; 1–2 mg/kg produces virtual complete inhibition of cyclo-oxygenase-dependant platelet aggregation.

Clopidrogel and ticlopidine

Ticlopidine and its chemical analogue, clopidrogel block the activation of platelets by ADP by selectively and irreversibly inhibiting the binding of ADP to its receptor on platelets and thereby inhibiting the ADP-dependent activation of the glycoprotein IIb/IIIa complex. Although only slightly more effective than aspirin, ticlopidine and clopidogrel show promise when combined with aspirin, probably because they block complementary pathways of platelet activation. Thus, the combination of aspirin and ticlopidine is superior to aspirin alone or to aspirin plus warfarin in patients undergoing coronary stent insertion. Despite its potential advantages, the widespread use of ticlopidine has been limited by an unacceptable side-effect profile, including diarrhoea, skin reactions and potentially fatal bone marrow suppression. Because of the potential adverse effects, haematological monitoring is necessary. Standard dose of ticlopidine is 250 mg twice daily for 2–4 weeks. Haematological monitoring is performed every 2 weeks and for at least 2 weeks after treatment cessation.

Clopidrogel

Clopidrogel is about six times as active as ticlopidine in inhibiting ADP-induced platelet aggregation inhuman platelets and has a better side-effect profile than ticlopidine. Dosage is 75mg daily usually for 4 weeks following coronary stent implantation with an initial loading dose of 300mg. Although it is not currently licensed for angioplasty/stenting most interventional centres are routinely using it.

Glycoprotein IIb/IIIa inhibitors

The activated glycoprotein IIb/IIIa receptor binds to a variety of ligands initiating platelet adhesion and aggregation resulting in the creation and propagation of thrombus. Based on this pathophysiology, specific inhibitors for the glycoprotein IIb/IIIa receptor have been developed. Those currently under investigation fall into three main categories:

- Monoclonal antibody Fab fragment to the glycoprotein IIb/IIIa receptor (abciximab).

- Peptide glycoprotein IIb/IIIa receptor antagonists (Integrilin).

- Non-peptide glycoprotein IIb/IIIa antagonists (lamifiban and tirofiban).

ReoPro or abciximab has been the most extensively studied in patients undergoing angioplasty. It is a potent, high-affinity, non-selective inhibitor of platelet aggregation and is an effective antithrombotic agent in acute myocardial ischaemic syndromes that require percutaneous coronary interventions. Abciximab plus aspirin is more effective than aspirin alone, and the addition of abciximab to aspirin and ticlopidine is more effective than aspirin and ticlopidine alone. Potential adverse effects include allergic reactions, thrombocytopenia and uncontrolled bleeding.

ReoPro is clinically effective when re-administered during percutaneous coronary intervention and is not associated with an increased risk of allergic or other hypersensitivity reactions.[15]

Dosage is 0.25 mg/kg IV bolus followed by 0.125 mg/kg/min continuous IV infusion. In the event of uncontrolled bleeding or thrombocytopenia, platelet transfusion is recommended.

Antithrombin agents

Heparin

Heparin is the most widely used antithrombin. The major effect of heparin is exerted via its interaction with antithrombin-III and thrombin in reducing thrombotic occlusions and major cardiac events in patients undergoing PTCA/stenting.

Heparin is used in combination with aspirin to prevent acute thrombotic closure during PTCA. A weight based dose, 70-100U/kg is administered IV initially with subsequent hourly boluses or infusion of heparin to maintain an activated clotting time (ACT) of > 200s during the procedure.

Low molecular weight heparin – use of low-molecular weight heparin in the angioplasty population does not appear to have a significant sustained benefit over unfractionated heparin.

Hirudin

Hirudin is a leech-derived peptide that binds directly with high affinity to several sites on thrombin and can inactivate clot-bound thrombin which heparin cannot do. However, the results to date with hirudin in the angioplasty population have shown no clear advantage over heparin.

CATHETER-BASED TREATMENTS FOR OTHER CARDIAC EMERGENCIES

Aortic balloon valvuloplasty

Percutaneous balloon valvuloplasty has been proposed as a less invasive means of treating aortic stenosis. It is, however, not an alternative to aortic valve replacement in adults.[16]

Method

Both antegrade and retrograde approaches have been described, the latter performed via puncture of the inter-atrial septum. The aortic valve is crossed with an extra stiff guidewire over which a dilation balloon is passed. Multiple inflation are performed until the properly sized balloon is fully inflated. Balloon dilatation improves the valvular cross-sectional area primarily by fracture of calcific deposits and splitting of fused commissures.

Indications

- Patients with aortic stenosis who are not candidates for surgical valve replacement but in whom balloon valvuloplasty would be expected to palliate severe symptoms or stabilize cardiogenic shock.

- Patients with aortic stenosis who are potentially suitable for definitive surgical treatment in the future but first require stabilization of aortic stenosis for urgent non-cardiac surgery.

Complications

Complications of aortic valvuloplasty include:

- High rates of restenosis.

- Aortic regurgitation.

- Leaflet avulsion.

- Aortic rupture.

- Ventricular perforation.

- Systemic embolization.

Percutaneous mitral balloon valvulolasty

Indications

- Percutaneous mitral balloon valvuloplasty provides substantial and sustained clinical benefit in selected patients with rheumatic mitral stenosis. It has been used with benefit to treat patients in acute pulmonary oedema and cardiogenic shock secondary to rheumatic mitral stenosis.[17]

- The technique has been used successfully to treat pulmonary oedema and right heart failure occurring secondary to mitral stenosis in pregnancy.

Method

The valve is usually approached in an antegrade direction via an interatrial septal puncture. The mechanism of improvement in the valve area is via splitting of the fused commissures.

Procedural outcome depends on the severity of four characteristics:

- Leaflet mobility.
- Valvular thickening.
- Subvalvular thickening.
- Valvular calcification.

Complications include:

- Leaflet tears or chordal or papillary rupture leading to mitral regurgitation.
- Ventricular perforation.
- Tamponade.
- Systemic embolization.

Transcatheter devices for post-infarction ventricular septal defect closure

Acute post-infarction ventricular septal rupture carries a high mortality rate. Transcatheter closure devices are an established method of treating selected congenital defects. The use of such devices for post-infarction VSD closure may provide short-term haemodynamic stabilization before urgent surgery, a bridging measure to allow myocardial strengthening by scarring before definitive surgery or a permanent alternative to primary or redo surgery.[18] Clinical experience is so far limited. Device migration has been the main complication of transcatheter closure.

Catheter-based treatment of acute aortic dissection

The objective of this treatment approach used to treat dissections that originate in the descending aorta is to seal the entry tear, promote thrombosis of the false lumen and stabilize the dissection using a catheter-delivered endovascular stent-graft. Catheter-based treatment of aortic dissection has been used in patients in whom the dissection originates in the descending aorta, whether or not the dissection involves retrograde extension into the ascending aorta. Following arteriographic evaluation of the entry tear, the stent graft is delivered via a transfemoral approach and is placed within the true lumen of the aorta. After the device is deployed, arteriography or intravascular ultrasonography is performed to confirm the position of the device relative to the entry tear. Initial results suggest that stent-graft coverage of the primary entry tear may be a promising new treatment for selected patients with acute aortic dissection.[19]

Further reading

Baim DS, Grossman W. Cardiac catheterization, angiography and intervention. 5th edn. Baltimore: Williams & Wilkins, 1996.

Roubin GS, Califf RM, O'Neil WW et al. Interventional Cardiovascular Medicine: Principles and Practice. Edinburgh: Churchill Livingstone, 1994.

References

1. Grines CL. Should thrombolysis or primary angioplasty be the treatment of choice for acute myocardial infarction? Primary angioplasty – the strategy of choice. N Engl J Med 1996; 335: 1313–17.

2. Stone GW, Grines CL, Browne KF et al. Predictors of in-hospital and 6-month outcome after acute myocardial infarction in the reperfusion era: the Primary Angioplasty in Myocardial Infarction (PAMI) trial. J Am Coll Cardiol 1995; 25: 310–17.

3. Nunn CM, O'Neil WW, Rothbaum D et al. Long-term outcome after primary angioplasty: report from the Primary Angioplasty in Myocardial Infarction (PAMI-I) trail. J Am Coll Cardiol 1999; 33: 640–6.

4. Wharton TP, McNamara NS, Fedele FA et al. Primary angioplasty for the treatment of acute myocardial infarction: experience at two community hospitals without cardiac surgery. J Am Coll Cardiol 1999; 33: 1257–65.

5. Ellis SG, van de Werf F, Ribeio da Silva E et al. Present status of rescue coronary angioplasty: Current polarization of opinion and randomized trials. J Am Coll Cardiol 1992; 19: 681–6.

6. Hochman JS, Sleeper LA, Webb JG et al. Early revacularization in acute myocardial infarction complicated by cardiogenic shock. 1999; 341: 625–34. N Eng J Med

7. Labinaz M, Ellis SG, Phillips HR et al. The role of angioplasty after successful thrombolysis for acute myocardial infarction. Coron Artery Dis 1994; 5: 399–406.

8. Halon DA, Flugelman MY, Merdler A *et al*. Long-term (10-year) outcome in patients with unstable angina pectoris treated by coronary balloon angioplasty. *J Am Coll Cardiol* 1998; **32**: 1603–9.

9. The EPIC Investigators. Use of a monoclonal antibody directed against the platelet glycoprotein IIb/IIIa receptor in high risk coronary angioplasty. *N Engl J Med* 1994; **330**: 956–61.

10. Pepine CJ, Holmes DR. Coronary artery stents – ACC Expert Consensus Document. *J Am Coll Cardiol* 1996; **28**: 782–94.

11. De Feyter PJ. Bailout coronary stenting: not always a foolproof safety net. *Am Heart J* 1999; **137**: 579–81.

12. Stone GW, Brodie BR, Griffin JJ *et al*. Prospective, multicentre study of safety and feasibility of primary stenting in acute myocardial infarction: in-hospital and 30-day results of the PAMI Stent Pilot Trial. *J Am Coll Cardiol* 1998; **31**: 23–30.

13. Stone GW, Claude-Morice M, Cox D *et al*. Predictors of six month event-free survival after mechanical reperfusion in acute myocardial infarction – the PAMI Stent Randomized Trial. *J Am Coll Cardiol* 1999; **33 (suppl. A)**: 379A.

14. Alexander JH, Harrington RA. Antiplatelet and antithrombin therapies in the acute coronary syndromes. *Curr Opin Cardiol* 1997; **12**: 427–37.

15. Tcheng JE, Kereiakes DJ, George BS *et al*. Safety of readministration of abciximab; interim results of the ReoPro readministration registry [R3]. *J Am Coll Cardiol* 1998; **31 (suppl. A)**: 55A.

16. Lewin RF, Dorros G, King JF *et al*. Percutaneous transluminal aortic valvuloplasty: acute outcome and follow-up of 125 patients. *J Am Coll Cardiol* 1989; **14**: 1210–17.

17. Goldman JH, Slade A, Clague J. Cardiogenic shock secondary to mitral stenosis treated by balloon mitral valvuloplasty. *Cathet Cardiovasc Diagn* 1998; **43**: 195–7.

18. Lee EM, Roberts DH, Walsh KP. Transcatheter closure of residual postmyocardial infarction ventricular septal defect with the Amplatz septal occluder. *Heart* 1998; **80**: 522–4.

19. Dake MD, Kato N, Scott Michael R *et al*. Endovascular stent-graft placement for the treatment of acute aortic dissection. *N Engl J Med* 1999; **340**: 1546–52.

11

CARDIAC ARREST

Cardiac arrest is cessation of effective circulation due to asystole, ventricular fibrillation (VF) and electromechanical dissociation (EMD) (electrical activity without cardiac output).

- Brain damage will occur within 4–6 min (unless protected by hypothermia). Therefore, this is the ultimate cardiac emergency.

- One of the truly landmark papers in the 20th century was that on closed chest cardiac resuscitation in 1960 by Kouwenhoven.

- This was the start of the modern concept of cardiopulmonary resuscitation (CPR).

This chapter will briefly review current guidelines for basic life support (BLS) and advanced life support (ALS) and discuss some of the controversies in resuscitation research. The practical aspects of BLS and ALS are not covered in detail as these are best learnt at formal resuscitation courses.

All hospital doctors should be proficient at CPR and should receive regular training/practice at BLS and ALS.

CAUSES

- Asystole is the first diagnosed rhythm in about 30% of cardiac arrest victims. In some, especially out-of-hospital arrests, this will be due to untreated VF (especially if bystander CPR has not been initiated). In hospital, asystole may be due to severe coronary artery disease and myocardial infarction. Occasionally hypoxia and other acute, severe medical conditions may result in asystolic arrest. Rarely asystole may be due to excess vagal stimulation or carotid sinus hypersensitivity.

- 'Sudden death' outside hospital is a major form of cardiac death. The majority of these are VF or pulseless ventricular tachycardia (VT) and are due to ischaemic heart disease. If untreated, all VF will degenerate into asystole. One study of > 1700 patients found that if the paramedics arrived within 4 min, 53% had VF/VT. With time the incidence of VF/VT decreased to 27% at 20 min.[1] Bystander CPR maintained VF.

EMD usually has a potentially reversible cause, e.g.:

- **H**ypovolaemia.
- **H**ypoxia.
- **H**yperkalaemia.
- **H**ypokalaemia.
- **H**ypothermia.
- **T**ension pneumothorax.
- **T**amponade.
- Drug **T**oxicity.
- **T**hromboembolism.

SURVIVAL

Overall, results are disappointing. Survival depends in part on the institution of bystander CPR and the time from arrest to defibrillation. Survival of up to 25% in out-of-hospital arrests is possible with rapid bystander CPR – survival is often higher for arrests in public than arrests at home.

One might expect survival from arrests in hospital to be better due to rapid availability of trained personnel and equipment but overall results are equally poor. This is due to the presence of other pathology than ischaemic heart disease in many of these patients. The exception is cardiac arrest due to VF in CCU for which survival is high because of immediate defibrillation – though many of these patients will not receive formal CPR.

FACTORS INCREASING SURVIVAL

- VF v asystole.
- Rapid CPR.
- Rapid defibrillation – survival of out-of-hospital arrest 43% if BLS < 4 min and defibrillation, < 8 min.[2]
- Short duration of CPR.
- Witnessed arrest.

- Bystander CPR if out-of-hospital.

- Defibrillation at scene if out-of-hospital.

- Effectiveness of CPR (see below).

- Skill and training of resuscitation personnel.

- Location of arrest in hospital – favourable if arrest in CCU, ICU or A&E. Although cardiac arrest under anaesthesia rare, these have highest resuscitation success rates.

BASIC LIFE SUPPORT (BLS) PROTOCOLS

Reference should be made to the latest guidelines as listed in further reading. This brief summary assumes two rescuers. In summary:

- First establish the need for intervention by feeling carotid pulse.

- Call for expert help.

- First rescuer – if no sign of respirations, assess and open airway by tilting head backwards and lifting jaw. Inflate lungs using equipment provided in your institution at a ratio of one breath/five cardiac compression (2:15 if only one rescuer).

- Second rescuer – if no signs of circulation, provide external cardiac massage (ECM) using two interlocked hands over lower third of sternum. Aim for cardiac compression rate of about 100/min.

- Monitor BLS for return of pulse and breathing.

- Remember – early BLS and defibrillation shown to improve outcome.

Exceptions to the above include a witnessed VF arrest in CCU where BLS need not be performed if defibrillation can be immediately performed (unless defibrillation unsuccessful!). A precordial thump may be attempted while defibrillator mobilized.

MECHANISMS OF ECM

- Original theory – heart squeezed between sternum and vertebral column with blood expelled with each compression. Relaxation 'sucks' blood back into the thorax. Some animal studies lend some credence to this theory.

- Thoracic pump theory – coughing during cardiac arrest can generate effective systolic pressures suggesting that high intrathoracic pressures can promote cardiac output. In this theory the heart serves as a conduit and increasing thoracic pressures during ECM expel blood out of the heart down a pressure gradient between intra- and extrathoracic vasculature.

CONTROVERSIES IN BLS/ECM

Awareness of the thoracic pump theory of cardiac output during ECM led to refinements that could be expected lead to increased output.

Active compression/decompression

A 'kitchen sink plunger' type of mechanism attached to the chest that improved ventricular filling and forward flow by 'sucking' blood into the chest has been investigated. However, a large trial has found no differences in outcome.[3]

Abdominal counterpulsation

Pressure on the abdominal aorta during ECM to improve filling of the heart again showed initial promise.

Pneumatic vest

Circumferential pressure on the thorax with a pneumatic system increases intrathoracic pressure and again showed initial promise.

However, the message from all these adjuncts to standard ECM is that non-supplant standard ECM at present.

Duration of compressions

Increasing the duration of compressions to about 50% of the ECM cycle is beneficial in animals and is a useful practical 'side-effect' of increasing the rate of compressions to about 100/min.

Open chest massage

Usefulness is limited to trauma and in the operating theatre especially during cardiac surgery. Such heroics do not lend themselves to routine performance by cardiac arrest teams. Similarly, placing the arrested patient onto cardiopulmonary bypass is limited mainly to cardiac surgery patients.

INFECTIOUS DISEASES

There is no doubt that fear of HIV transmission is limiting the application of BLS techniques by lay bystanders. This is despite education that HIV has not been reported to be transmitted by saliva contact.

Nevertheless, it is prudent to take precautions (TB and viruses such as herpes can definitely be transmitted during BLS). All hospital personnel should have access to devices such as pocket masks, etc. that should negate the necessity for 'mouth-to-mouth' resuscitation.

However, this has no impact on the fear of lay bystanders. It has, therefore, been suggested[4] that lay CPR should concentrate on ECM only, i.e. no mouth-to-mouth, particularly if there is only one rescuer. The rationale is based on animal studies showing that ventilation during CPR is not as important as ECM.

Clinical studies clearly show:

- Bystander ventilation only → no ↑ survival; cf. no resuscitation.

- Bystander ECM only → ↑ survival.

- No further ↑ survival with both ECM and ventilation.

ADVANCED LIFE SUPPORT (ALS) PROTOCOLS

BLS alone will rarely result in successful resuscitation. The purpose of BLS is to maintain organ blood flow until techniques can be applied to restore spontaneous circulation.

Summary of ALS principles:

- Maintain CPR/BLS.

- Precordial thump if VF witnessed followed by immediate defibrillation if necessary.

- Verify rhythm – defibrillate with 200, 200 then 360 joules. Take care with paddle positions. Note: 80% of successful defibrillations occur in first three shocks.

- Appropriate IV access (see below).

- Ensure oxygenation and intubation if appropriate personnel present. Oxygenate before attempting intubation and avoid prolonged attempts without re-oxygenation.

- In general, patients do not die of failure to intubate; they die of failure to oxygenate. However, intubation is probably worthwhile if only to protect against aspiration of stomach contents.

- Drug administration is simplified in latest guidelines (see further reading). Basically consists of 1 mg adrenaline every 3 min. Atropine, 3 mg, may be given **once** in asystole.

- Be aware of potentially reversible causes of EMD (see Causes).

Immediate transthoracic external pacing is recommended in some protocols for management of asystole but does not occupy a position of priority in the European guidelines (possibly due to lack of routine access to the equipment).

DRUG CONTROVERSIES IN ALS

Adrenaline

Boluses of 1 mg adrenaline IV are currently the recommended drug of choice in almost all circumstances in cardiac arrest. However, this is despite a lack of convincing clinical evidence showing that adrenaline improves survival or neurological outcome. Certainly there are animal studies showing improved myocardial and cerebral blood flow and survival, but patient studies are conflicting.

The rationale for the administration of adrenaline includes:

- α vasoconstricting effect raising coronary and cerebral perfusion pressures. This improves the chances of successful defibrillation in VF.

- The β_1 effect may coarsen fine VF or promote VF in asystole. Its positive inotropic effects are of lesser importance.

- Positive chronotropic effects may be useful if bradycardia occurs.

Because of favourable animal studies higher doses have been tried (up to 10 mg) but have not led to improved survival. In fact, disappointingly, neither 'normal'- nor 'high'-dose adrenaline produced improved survival compared with placebo in a recent study.[5]

Vasopressin

Disenchantment with clinical results from the use of adrenaline has resulted in other vasoconstrictors being investigated. For example, in a randomized controlled study the use of 40 μg vasopressin (a non-catecholamine vasopressor) produced increased 24-h survival compared with 1mg adrenaline.[6] Although only a small study, these results are encouraging, but it is too early for widespread adoption of vasopressin in ALS.

Atropine

The rationale for the use of atropine comes from studies showing high endogenous catecholamine levels during cardiac arrest (implying presumably a limited effect from additional exogenous catecholamines) and a relatively high vagal tone.[7] However, atropine administration has not been shown to improve survival from cardiac arrest and its role is currently secondary to that of adrenaline.

Calcium chloride

Although calcium salts have a positive inotropic action, its use has not been shown to improve survival in cardiac arrest. Use now should be restricted to hyperkalaemia, hypocalcaemia or arrests secondary to overdosage of calcium-blocking drugs. There is also concern that high blood levels of calcium could precipitate coronary spasm in patients with ischaemic heart disease and also potentially increase cerebral damage during periods of ischaemia. For similar reasons dextrose-containing fluids should be avoided during cardiac arrest.

Sodium bicarbonate

No longer routinely administrated due to concerns about the production of a hyperosmolar state, 'overshoot' alkalosis (detrimental effect on oxyhaemoglobin dissociation curve-limiting oxygen release at the tissues) and hypernatraemia. The use of bicarbonate is best reserved for prolonged resuscitation, i.e. pH < 7.1, where the myocardium may be directly compromised. Most useful in hyperkalaemic arrest or arrest following tricyclic antidepressant overdosage.

Antiarrhythmic administration

The usefulness of many anti-arrhythmic drugs during cardiac arrest is limited by their negative inotropic properties.

- Lignocaine is currently widely used during prolonged VF arrests and to prevent recurrence of VF. Although controversial this use is supported by studies showing improved outcome from sustained VF arrests.[8] Interestingly, lignocaine is known to increase defibrillation threshold.

- Bretylium lowers defibrillation threshold and is beneficial in sustained VF. Convincing evidence for improved **survival**, however, is lacking.

- The cardiac depressant effect of amiodarone is relatively mild and well tolerated. An important randomized, controlled trial of out-of-hospital cardiac arrest has been presented at a major scientific meeting. The ARREST trial found that a 300g bolus of amiodarone improved survival to hospital compared with placebo.[9] If this is substantiated by further studies and the improved survival translates to improved survival to discharge, it will have important implications.

ROUTE OF DRUG ADMINISTRATION

- Initial administration of drugs is best via good peripheral venous access. Drug injections should be well flushed.

- With prolonged resuscitation central venous catheterization may be appropriate **if** performed by experienced personnel (pneumothorax from unskilled central venous attempts is counterproductive!). Many find it difficult to catheterize a central vein during ECM – but this is not an indication to stop CPR.

- If no vascular access possible, adrenaline, lignocaine and atropine may all be given via the endotracheal tube at twice the normal dose, preferably diluted to 10 ml. Blood levels of drugs given by the endotracheal route are unpredictable.

- Intracardiac injection is no longer recommended due to the potential for trauma.

MONITORING EFFECTIVENESS OF CPR

Cardiac output only, at best, 10–30% of normal during CPR. Flow is especially poor to organs below the diaphragm. Presence of a carotid pulse is not a reliable **quantitative** indicator of cardiac output. Pupillary responses during CPR are not helpful – beware of the effects of adrenaline and atropine.

Indicators of effective CPR:

- Arterial pressure tracing if arterial line *in situ* – especially with diastolic > 40 mmHg.

- Measured CO_2 in expired gas or end tidal CO_2. Measured with simple hand-held device attachable to breathing circuit. Chemical indicators provide a semiquantitative indicator of pCO_2. Increases with CPR indicate increasing cardiac output and pulmonary artery blood flow and a likely successful outcome.

Indicators of ineffective CPR:

- As above, lack of increasing end tidal CO_2 predicts a poor outcome.

- Worsening metabolic acidosis indicates poor tissue blood flow. Venous pH may be more useful than arterial as will better reflect the acid–base state of the tissues.

COMPLICATIONS OF CPR

- Ineffective ECM, including situations where circulation has been re-established but neurological outcome is poor because of relatively ineffective ECM.

- Stomach distension, potentially leading to regurgitation and pulmonary aspiration.

- (Arguably fear of this complication is one of the main reasons for endotracheal intubation of the patient.)

- Rib and sternal fractures.

- Laceration of liver and other abdominal organs has been reported.

- Complications of central vascular access, e.g. pneumothorax.

- Potential pro-arrthythmic effects of drugs administered. Certainly, tachycardia following successful resuscitation is widespread.

- Complications of defibrillation – including burns to patient, shocks to operator (no deaths reported) and explosion of GTN patches. It is recommended that patches are removed and to keep paddles 10–15 cm away from pacemakers.

NEUROLOGICAL OUTCOME

- One study found that an arrest time before resuscitation (or 'down time') > 6 min or CPR time > 15 min **always** produced neurological impairment. However, down times < 6 min and CPR times of < 30 min resulted in satisfactory neurological recovery in 50% of patients.[10] One implication of this is to limit resuscitation attempts to < 15 min where down time is > 6 min.

- Scoring systems have been developed using various clinical signs to try and predict the likelihood of neurological recovery but, unfortunately, none is sufficiently accurate to enable definite pronouncements on prognosis to be made in advance.

- EEG monitoring may occasionally be useful and improves the ability to predict outcome.

- Many believe that lack of corneal reflexes or pupillary light reflexes after 24 h indicates a uniformly poor outcome.

Some points from the literature:

- Most who recover show rapid improvement in the first 24–48 h.

- Coma persisting > 4 h makes neurological damage more likely.

- Long duration of coma (especially > 4 days) leads to very poor outcome.

POST-RESUSCITATION CARE

- Depends on underlying cause of the arrest. Specific causes may obviously need specific treatment.

- VF associated with MI – treatment largely that of MI.

- In the USA many patients undergo emergency cardiac catheterization with aggressive reperfusion attempted in some centres.

- Control blood glucose – hyperglycaemia is associated with a worse neurological outcome.

- BP autoregulation is impaired – avoid hypo- or hypertension.

- Occasionally patients have a low cardiac output and develop multiple organ failure. The myocardial dysfunction is suggestive of some degree of 'myocardial stunning'. Animal studies support the use of dobutamine.

- Drug therapy to improve neurological outcome is still experimental – much interest, so far fruitless, in the use of calcium blockers.

- Intracranial pressure is not usually increased. Recent research confirms that, as for head injuries, routine hyperventilation in an attempt at 'cerebral salvage' can **lower** cerebral blood flow.

- Many centres offer IPPV and ICU care in an effort to optimize haemodynamics and oxygenation but there is no evidence that this approach improves outcome in this rather depressing clinical situation.

TRAINING

- In general, studies showing best survival in out-of-hospital arrests are those in which early bystander CPR is initiated. Therefore, community wide programmes of BLS modelled on Seattle and Belgian experience would seem important.

- Unfortunately poor knowledge among doctors is still a problem.[11] This is despite the studies clearly demonstrating that patient survival varies with knowledge of correct management as well as availability of equipment. All doctors (indeed all healthcare personnel) should undergo training and practice of CPR skills. The majority of hospitals now have full time resuscitation training officers for this purpose. Six-monthly re-instruction has been shown to maintain adequate skills.

Further reading

Advanced Life Support Working Group of the European Resuscitation Council. The 1998 European Resuscitation Council guidelines for adult advanced life support. *Br Med J* 1998; **316**: 1863–9.

Ballew KA. Recent advances: cardiopulmonary resuscitation. *Br Med J* 1997; **314**: 1462–5.

Basic Life Support Working Group of the European Resuscitation Council. The 1998 European Resuscitation Council guidelines for adult single rescuer basic life support. *Br Med J* 1998; **316**: 1870–6.

References

1. Herlitz J, Ekstrom L, Wennerblom B *et al.* Type of arrhythmia at EMS arrival on scene in out-of-hospital cardiac arrest in relation to interval from collapse and whether a bystander initiated CPR. *Am J Emerg Med* 1996; **14**: 119–23.

2. Eizenberg MS, Bergner L, Hallstrom A. Cardiac resuscitation in the community: Importance of rapid provision and implications for program planning. *J Am Med Assoc* 1979; **241**: 1905–9.

3. Stiell IG, Hebert PC, Wells GA *et al.* The Ontario trial of active compression–decompression for in-hospital and prehospital cardiac arrests. *J Am Med Assoc* 1996; **275**: 1417–23.

4. Berg RA, Wilcoxson D, Hilwig RW *et al.* The need for ventilatory support during bystander CPR. *Ann Emerg Med* 1995; **26**: 342–50.

5. Woodhouse SP, Cox S, Boyd P *et al.* High dose and standard dose adrenaline do not alter survival, compared with placebo. *Resuscitation* 1995; **30**: 243–9.

6. Lindner KH, Dirks B, Strohmenger HU *et al.* Randomized comparison of epinephrine and vasopressin in patients with out-of-hospital ventricular fibrillation. *Lancet* 1997; **349**: 535–7.

7. Little RA, Frayn KN, Randall PE *et al.* Plasma catecholamines in patients with acute myocardial infarction and in cardiac arrest. *Q J Med* 1985; **214**: 133–40.

8. Herlit J, Ekstrom L, Wennerblom B *et al.* Lidocaine in out-of-hospital ventricular fibrillation. Does it improve survival? *Resuscitation* 1997; **33**: 199–205.

9. Kern KB. Drug therapy in advanced cardiac life support. *Curr Opin Crit Care* 1998; **4**: 161–4.

10. Abramson NS, Safar P, Detre KM *et al.* Neurologic recovery after cardiac arrest: effect of duration of ischaemia. *Crit Care Med* 198; **13**: 930–1.

11. Tham KY, Evans RJ, Rubython EJ, Kinnaird TD. Management of ventricular fibrillation by doctors in cardiac arrest teams. *Br Med J* 1994; **309**: 1408–9.

12

ACUTE MYOCARDIAL INFARCTION AND UNSTABLE ANGINA: ACUTE CORONARY SYNDROMES

Acute myocardial infarction (MI) and unstable angina are among the commonest reasons for acute medical admission. Previously a clear distinction was drawn between these apparently separate entities based on biochemical and electrocardiographic markers. However, as more has become known about their pathogenesis it has become clear that a continuum of disease exists from stable angina through unstable angina, to non-Q-wave MI and finally to transmural or Q-wave MI. Despite this, it is still valuable to discuss Q-wave MI separately from unstable angina and non-Q-wave MI, mainly because the treatment options differ significantly.

ACUTE MYOCARDIAL INFARCTION – Q-WAVE

A Q-wave MI occurs when there is a sustained severe reduction in myocardial blood flow sufficient to cause irreversible damage through the full thickness of the ventricular wall, although recently it has been shown that the presence or absence of Q-waves does not reliably predict transmural infarction.[1] This is almost exclusively caused by acute thrombosis of the supplying vessel. The process of thrombosis is complex, usually involving plaque rupture, platelet adhesion and activation, and thrombin formation.

Clinical presentation

- Pain – the most consistent feature. Typically this is described as the most severe pain ever experienced. It is usually present for > 30 min, centrally or left-sided in location and tight or crushing in character. It often radiates to the neck and/or arm and typically does not respond to sublingual glyceryl trinitrate. In certain subgroups, in particular the elderly and in patients with diabetic neuropathy, pain may not be experienced.

- Breathlessness – often accompanies the pain and may be due to the myocardial ischaemia itself or be a manifestation of acute pulmonary oedema.

- Sympathetic and parasympathetic overactivity – often leads to vomiting, sweating, dizziness, palpitations and feeling clammy.

- Typically symptoms have no obvious precipitating factor but in a proportion of patients a MI occurs following anxiety or strenuous activity. There is also a well-documented circadian variation with a peak occurring in the early morning (06:00–09:00 hours). This is probably related to increases in catecholamines and platelet aggregability.

- Regrettably one of the commonest presentations of acute MI is sudden death, where the MI has usually been associated with a sudden fatal ventricular arrhythmias. Of MI, 50% may present this way.

DIAGNOSIS OF MI

Electrocardiogram (ECG)

The initial ECG is regarded as being diagnostic in about 60% of patients, abnormal but non-diagnostic in 25% and normal in 15%. Sensitivity can be increased to 95% by serial recording of ECG.

The classic diagnosis of acute MI is based on the appearance of the T-wave and ST segment.

- Usually the T-wave changes are the first to occur and include inversion, flattening, 'hyperacute' changes (a peaked T-wave appears to start its upward slope immediately following the S-wave). The latter should not be confused with the normal appearance of 'high-takeoff', where the T-wave appears to begin from a point higher than the iso-electric line and may have a 'slurred upstroke'.

- This is followed by ST segment changes, elevation by ≥ 0.1 mV in two or more limb leads, or ≥ 0.2 mV in two or more contiguous precordial leads. Occasionally, ST depression can occur.

- Often ST depression is seen in leads that are 'opposite' to those showing ST elevation, but it can occur in patients who have sustained an isolated true posterior MI. In this situation the ECG shows widespread ST depression across the anterior precordial leads in association with a prominent R-wave in lead V1 (figure 1).

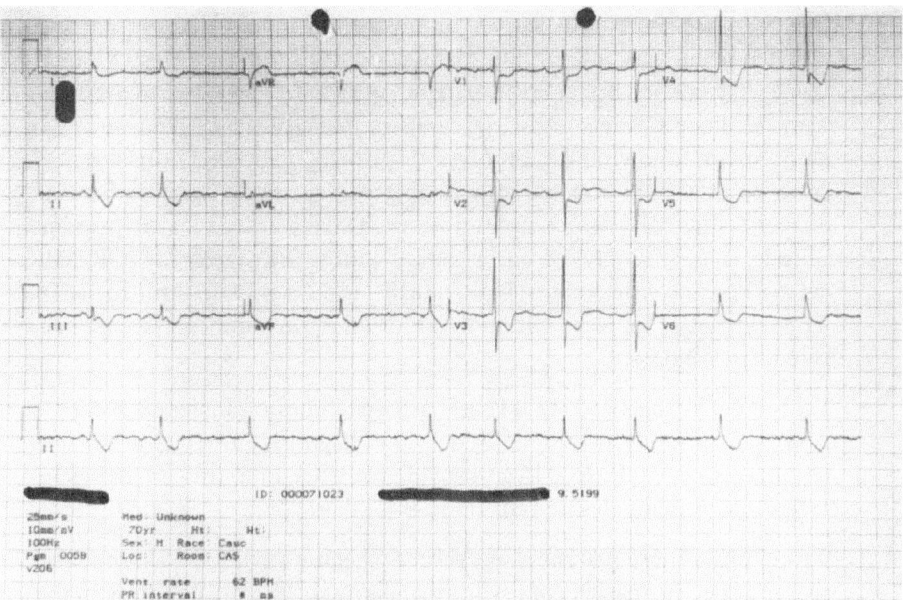

Figure 1. ECG showing changes consistent with a true posterior myocardial infarction (prominent R wave in lead V1, widespread ST segment depression in the anterior precordial leads). The patient is also in atrial fibrillation.

- Q-waves can be present on the presenting ECG, even in the earliest stages of infarction, but usually they develop later and persist indefinitely, particularly if reperfusion does not occur.

- New left bundle branch block (LBBB) is regarded as being indicative of severe widespread myocardial damage. It is often not possible to be certain if the LBBB is new as a previous ECG may not be available. In this situation diagnosis relies on the clinical history of the presenting chest pain and on the patient's history of previous MI (it may be more likely that the changes are old if the patient has had severe myocardial injury in the past).

The position of the ECG changes gives prognostic information as this often defines the proportion of the myocardium at risk. In order of decreasing degree of muscle damage, new LBBB indicates a large area of myocardial necrosis, followed by anterior ST elevation, followed by inferior ST elevation. However, this should only be taken as a general guide as some inferior MI can be associated with extensive infarction.

Cardiac enzymes

- Creatine kinase (CK) – CK is released following muscle damage and for years has been the main biochemical marker of infarction. Its use, however, has limitations as it is found in non-myocardial muscle and elevated levels can be found in many conditions without MI. The total CK level may not be raised in patients who have sustained myocardial damage. Total CK levels give a reliable estimate of the extent of muscle damage, but following thrombolysis or primary angioplasty this is not as accurate as CK is released more rapidly. For these reasons the iso-enzyme, CK-MB, which is almost exclusively found in myocardial muscle, is increasingly recommended as a more sensitive assay (CK-MB >6mg/l or catalytic activity higher than local diagnostic limit for MI). These enzymes increase within 4–6 h of infarction and can remain elevated for 3–4 days.

• Lactate dehydrogenase (LDH) and aspartate aminotransferase (AST) – AST is now rarely routinely used in the diagnosis of MI as it has few advantages over CK. LDH can provide evidence of a 'missed' MI as its levels may remain elevated for up to 8–14 days.

• Troponins – these markers have recently been shown to be more sensitive and specific markers of myocardial damage. Their use is more in the management of acute coronary syndromes or unstable angina.

Echocardiography and isotope perfusion scanning

• Both these imaging modalities can provide evidence of acute MI, but their use is not recommended as therapeutic decisions may be delayed. They may be helpful in cases where diagnostic uncertainty exists.

TREATMENT

There is no other area of medicine that has been researched in as much detail or included as many patients in clinical trials than the treatment of acute MI. It is beyond the scope of this chapter to discuss in detail all the trial results; however, a summary of the recommendations will be presented.

Reperfusion therapy

The goal of all therapies to treat MI is to provide rapid, complete and sustainable reperfusion of the infarcting myocardium. Although it may seem obvious, it is important to state that this can only be achieved by having an 'open' artery following the therapy. There are two main ways of achieving this end: pharmacological, by thrombolysis, and mechanical, by percutaneous transluminal coronary angioplasty (PTCA) (see Chapter 10).

Thrombolysis

- Administration of a thrombolytic agent to a patient with a MI is a medical emergency. It has been conclusively proven that delays in therapy cost lives. For each hour of delay from symptom onset, estimates of lives lost/1000 patients treated vary between 1.6 and 5.[2,3] Practically speaking, this means that thrombolysis should be administered with the minimum 'door-to-needle' time usually in an emergency room setting.

- Thrombolysis should only be administered to patients presenting with a history compatible with an acute MI who fulfil the ECG criteria mentioned above. It has never been proven that treatment of ST depression or non-Q-wave MI benefit from thrombolysis. In fact there are data to suggest that thrombolysis in these patients may actually worsen prognosis, probably due to the procoagulant effect seen following thrombolysis.[2] There is one potential exception to this rule as patients with true posterior MI may benefit.[4]

- There are currently many available thrombolytic drugs, although in the UK only two agents are widely used: streptokinase (SK) and recombinant tissue plasminogen activator (r-tPA). SK has the advantages of low cost, many years of experience of use and relative ease of administration. It can produce a mortality rate reduction of between 18 and 23%. Correspondingly r-tPA is slightly more complicated to administer and is much more expensive. Its advantages over SK were proven in the Global Utilisation of Streptokinase and Tissue Plasminogen Activator for Occluded Coronary Arteries (GUSTO–1) trial. An 'accelerated' regimen (> 1.5 h) produced a 15% reduction in mortality rate at 30 days in comparison with SK therapy. However, maximum benefit was seen in those with larger infarcts. Consequently it is common practice to give SK to small inferior infarcts, and r-tPA to anterior and extensive inferior infarcts. Newer, as yet not widely available, agents may have the benefit of single-bolus administration.

- Late therapy beyond 12 h after symptom onset does not provide any mortality rate benefit,[5] although it is possible that patients with ongoing chest pain and progressive elevation of ST-segments may derive some beneficial effect.

- There is no upper age limit for thrombolysis. The older population is not well represented in thrombolytic trials because of the increased risk of intracerebral haemorrhage with thrombolytic therapy. But conversely it is the elderly who have potentially the most to gain as they have the highest mortality rate from acute MI.

- Repeat thrombolysis is indicated if there is evidence of repeated infarction with re-elevation of ST segments. SK can be re-administered provided it is < 5 days (or at least 6 months and probably longer) since the previous administration, although if the interval is very short (a few hours) it may be best to give r-tPA as this gives better reperfusion rates.

- There are contraindications to thrombolytic therapy. However, when interpreting these the potential risk–benefit ratio for each patient needs to be assessed. For example, one might be more inclined to thrombolize an anterior MI (where there is a larger proportion of myocardium at risk) with a relative contraindication than an inferior infarct with a similar contraindication. Widely accepted contraindications to thrombolysis are presented in table 1.

- It is necessary to administer IV heparin when using r-tPA and to continue an IV infusion for at least 24 h following thrombolysis hopefully to maintain artery patency. SK has a longer half-life, which requires no adjunctive therapy.

- It is likely that treatment with a thrombolytic agent can save up to 30 lives/1000 patients treated.[6]

Mechanical reperfusion

Based on the information from the thrombolytic trials, it became clear that an open infarct-related artery conferred both significant mortality and morbidity rate benefits.[7] However, it was also clear that thrombolysis was failing in a high proportion of cases, as up to 40–50% of IRA did not show normal flow after thrombolysis.[8] The role of catheter-based techniques as an adjunct or alternative to thrombolysis is fully discussed in Chapter 10.

Currently it is not possible in the UK to offer such a service in all hospitals and transfer to centres with facilities may delay reperfusion. Therefore, for the majority of patients thrombolysis will still be the mainstay of therapy.

Table 1 – Contraindications to thrombolysis

Absolute	Relative
Active bleeding	Recent trauma or surgery > 2 weeks
Recent trauma or surgery < 2 weeks	Chronic severe hypertension
Prolonged CPR	Active peptic ulcer
Pregnancy	History of CVA
Suspected aortic dissection	Current use of anticoagulants
History of haemorrhagic CVA	Prior exposure to SK within 6–9 months if SK proposed once more
Previous allergic reaction to the proposed thrombolytic agent	

Certain subgroups of patients should, however, be considered for mechanical reperfusion and these include patients with cardiogenic shock due to a MI, patients who have on-going ischaemic chest pain following thrombolysis and patients with contraindications to thrombolysis. The contraindication to thrombolysis is usually due to as a result of an increased bleeding risk, and the perceived idea is that angioplasty offers lower risks in this area. The use of peri-procedural heparin and very potent IV and oral anti-platelet agents makes this distinction somewhat less absolute. As a general rule it is best to discuss relevant patients on an individual basis with the interventional centre.

Adjunctive medical therapy

Aspirin

Aspirin is extremely important as an anti-platelet agent in acute MI. Its benefits have become so well known that it is almost always given by paramedical and nursing staff before admission. Its benefits were proven in the International Study of Infarct Survival 2 (ISIS–2) trial, where 20 lives were saved/1000 treated.[9] The benefits are additive to those of thrombolysis. Aspirin should be administered as a dispersible 300 mg tablet as soon as a MI is suspected and 75–150 mg daily is probably sufficient thereafter.

β-Blockers

The benefits of IV β-blockers were first conclusively proven in the ISIS–1 trial and in the metoprolol in acute myocardial infarction (MIAMI) trial.[10] A total of six lives was saved/1000 treated. Both trials were conducted in the prethrombolytic era and their use has declined, mainly because of the fear of inducing bradyarrhythmia and left ventricular dysfunction. Their early use can paradoxically reduce the deleterious tachycardia often associated with MI and they reduce the incidence of ventricular arrhythmias and ventricular rupture. Consequently, it is recommended that atenolol 5 mg bolus IV should be administered as soon as possible following infarction (without delaying thrombolysis) to all patients who do not have a bradycardia, hypotension or pulmonary oedema. A further 5 mg bolus should be administered unless heart rate falls to < 60 beats/min, blood pressure (BP) drops or heart block ensues. Following the IV dose, oral β-blockade should be commenced and probably continued long-term as they do reduce the incidence of reinfarction and sudden death.[11]

Calcium channel blockers

This group of agents has been studied for some time post-myocardial infarction. There is some information that diltiazem and verapamil may be beneficial, but data are not conclusive. The shorter-acting dihydropyridine group agent nifedipine may have a deleterious effect. The routine use of these agents post-MI can not be recommended, except for symptom relief.

Nitrates

Nitrates are useful for relief of symptoms but do not provide any mortality rate benefit. There is a growing trend to treat patients who have a high BP on admission with nitrates to lower the BP and then proceed with thrombolysis. While this may be successful, it is much better to lower the BP in such a way as to provide prognostic benefit by giving an IV dose of a β-blocker.

Potassium channel openers

Nicorandil is the only agent of this class currently available. Once again it is useful for symptomatic relief, but is not used in the routine treatment of MI.

Angiotensin-converting enzyme inhibitors (ACE I)

Oral ACE inhibition is probably beneficial in the majority of patients presenting with a MI, both when started early or slightly later. However, the maximum benefits are seen with those who have had more extensive myocardial damage. The benefits have been well proven by multiple trials and five to 40 lives can be saved/1000 patients treated dependant on the treatment group. Current recommendations vary, but consideration should be given to treating all patients for 6 weeks initially and continuing in all patients with evidence of significant myocardial damage, i.e. clinical heart failure or echocardiographic evidence of LV dysfunction.

Cholesterol-lowering agents

Acute treatment of hyperlipidaemia has no short-term benefit; however, patients are often at their most receptive immediately post-MI and intervening on an elevated cholesterol with drug therapy at this stage may result in better compliance. It must be remembered that cholesterol levels will drop within 12–24 h of MI; consequently it is common policy to request lipids on the admission blood sample. Therapy with statins has now been conclusively shown to benefit the vast majority of patients with ischaemic heart disease and with elevated cholesterol levels.

Other agents

It is of paramount importance that any patient presenting with a MI has their pain and anxiety relieved as soon as possible with judicious use of opioids. But it must be borne in mind that the opioids do not provide significant anti-ischaemic benefits and attention should always be paid to the relief of ischaemia with the above-mentioned agents.

Complications

Heart failure (see Chapter 14)

Heart failure post-MI is a poor prognostic indicator. It may be due to left ventricular dysfunction, which is irreversible because of myocardial necrosis or reversible because of a temporary 'stunning' of the myocardium. Stunned myocardium is at least partially viable and usually recovers its function after a short period. ACE I and diuretic therapy should be used and the dose of ACE I should be quickly titrated up to the maximum tolerated dose.

Cardiogenic shock (see Chapter 13)

This is also a poor prognostic indicator as it almost always indicates severe myocardial damage. Supportive therapy with inotropic support is indicated and invasive monitoring with a pulmonary artery (PA) catheter can help its use. Occasionally the use of intra-aortic balloon counterpulsation (IABP) or coronary intervention may be indicated.

Heart block

Any degree of heart block can occur following MI. It is more common with inferior infarction as this is usually caused by right coronary occlusion and the atrioventricular node usually receives blood from this artery. When heart block occurs in association with anterior infarction, it is an ominous finding and usually indicates extensive myocardial damage. With the exception of first-degree heart block and perhaps episodic Wenkebach, all patients with heart block following MI should have a temporary pacing wire placed at the apex of the RV. In experienced hands this is a quick and safe procedure, but the commonest error made is in failing to secure the wire appropriately with potentially catastrophic results.

Arrhythmias

This is dealt with in more detail in Chapter 15, but many tachyarrythmias occur following a MI. As with all arrhythmias it is important to correct any electrolyte abnormalities. Wherever possible it is best to try to deal with them using β-blockers, perhaps using sotalol, which has class III anti-arrhythmic activity. When this is not possible or inappropriate, digoxin, amiodarone and lignocaine are the most commonly used. The latter is often useful in ventricular tachycardia, but it is negatively inotropic and should be used for the minimum period possible. Cardioversion should be used without delay in all haemodynamically compromising arrhythmias and in those not responding to medical therapy. Routine suppression of ventricular ectopics is contraindicated.

Others

- Ventricular perforation is often a premortem event, although if the perforation is contained by the pericardium a pseudo-aneurysm may ensue. Therapy is almost universally futile.

- Acute mitral regurgitation (MR) and ventricular septal defect are discussed in Chapter 17.

- Mural thrombus may develop adjacent to an area of hypokinetic myocardium. This may remain in position or embolize to the rest of the circulation. It is often diagnosed on echocardiography incidentally, but any embolic phenomena in a patient who has had a recent MI should be scanned. Formal anticoagulation should be instituted if confirmed.

• A LV aneurysm may develop late following MI and is a potential source for thrombus formation, persistent heart failure and ventricular arrhythmias. Its presence worsens LV function, and surgical repair is often carried out at the same time as coronary artery bypass surgery (CABG).

Right ventricular infarction

RV infarction warrants special mention because of the way in which damage to the RV produces a specific haemodynamic effect. RV infarction is very common, complicating up to 50% of inferior infarctions, most posterior infarcts and occasional anterior infarcts. It is poorly diagnosed as a RV chest lead (V4R) is not routinely performed (figure 2). Fortunately only 50% of RV infarcts produce haemodynamic effects. Management is discussed in Chapter 13.

The presence of RV infarction results in a dramatic deterioration in prognosis (up to 30% mortality rate); however, correctly managed RV infarction is survivable and the long-term prognosis is purely dependent on the degree of LV damage.

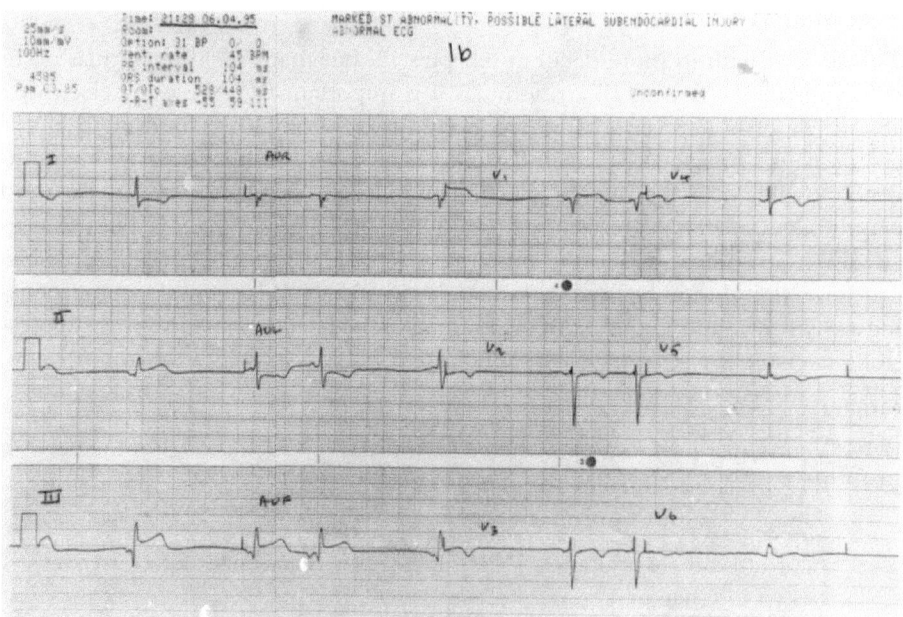

Figure 2a. ECG showing acute inferior myocardial infarction with ST elevation and Q waves in leads II, III and aVF. The patient is also developing a nodal rhythm.

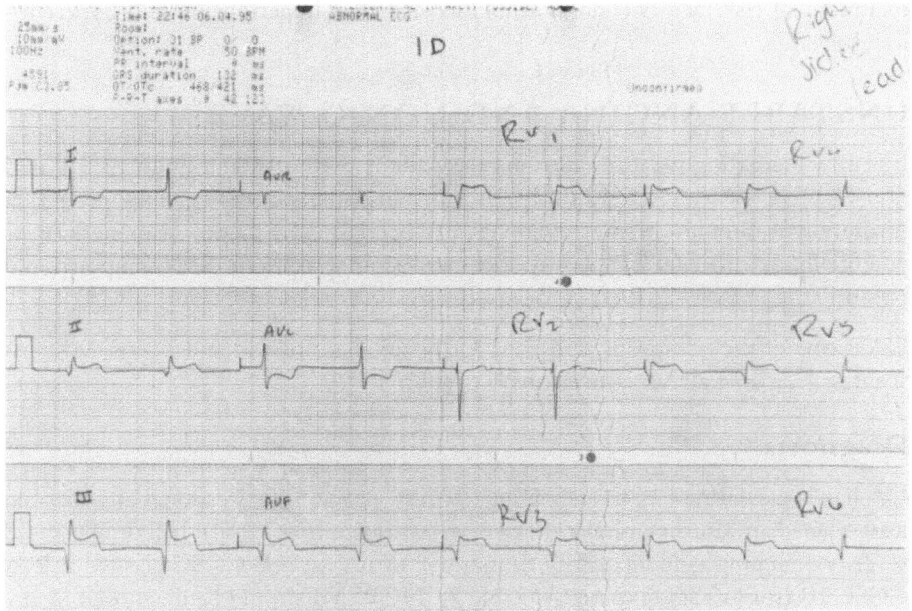

Figure 2b. Repeat ECG recording right-sided leads in the same patient showing ST elevation in RV3–6. The patient has had an inferior myocardial infarction complicated by right ventricular infarction. The patient is now in a nodal rhythm.

Post-myocardial infarction management

Any patient who develops recurrent ischaemic chest pain following initial treatment is in a poor prognostic group, with both higher mortality and reinfarction rates. Attention must focus on the detection and treatment of repeat infarction, but in those who do not reinfarct the management must be along the lines of unstable angina (see below).

In all patients who have had a MI it is mandatory to perform an assessment of the risk of that patient undergoing a further ischaemic event, unless their co-morbid condition does not permit. In the UK this usually involves an exercise or pharmacological stress test. Patients at higher risk are those who have a poor exercise time, develop ischaemic chest pain early and who develop significant ST-segment changes. Patients who are in one of these high-risk groups or who continue to experience chest pain are usually advised to have coronary angiography followed by revascularization, if appropriate.

Aside from the purely medical aspects of post-MI care, it is also very important to provide the patient with psychological support and advice as well as assistance in the return to as full a life as possible. These aims are most often met in the structured rehabilitation programmes now available in most hospitals. Part of this rehabilitation process is to reduce the patient's risk factors for recurrent events by treatment of risk factors such as smoking, diabetes, hypertension and hypercholesterolaemia.

UNSTABLE ANGINA AND NON-Q-WAVE MI

It is now increasingly common to discuss patients with unstable angina (UA) and non-Q-wave (NQW) MI as a similar group. This largely stems form the proof that thrombolytic therapy in these patients has been shown to not be beneficial or potentially detrimental.[12] There is also increasing agreement that therapy should be similar.

UA is one of the commonest reasons for hospital admission and NQW MI constitutes > 30% of all MI admissions.[13]

Diagnosis

UA has been defined as having angina at rest, new onset exertional angina of at least Canadian Cardiovascular Society Classification (CCSC) III, or increased severity of angina as indicated by an increase in at least one CCSC class to at least CCSC III (for CCSC grading, see table 2). NQW MI should be diagnosed in any patient whose cardiac enzymes are raised without the evidence of acute Q-wave MI, as discussed previously. Often this is accompanied by ST depression or T-wave inversion; however, a NQW MI does not have to have ECG changes present, provided the enzyme rise is definitely of cardiac origin.

As described above, the diagnosis of UA is predominantly clinical. However, troponin (T or I) estimation is now being used to stratify risk in these patients. An elevated level of troponin-T >0.1mg/l or positive qualitative troponin-T test is predictive of future MI and mortality rate.[14]

Pathogenesis

The mechanism of these acute coronary syndromes is complex but similar to acute MI in that it most usually involves plaque disruption. This leads to an acute reduction in coronary blood flow in contrast to the situation in stable angina, where increases in myocardial oxygen demand outstrip the ability of a stenosed coronary artery to supply it. In UA it is likely that there is transient (10–20 min) occlusion of a coronary artery accompanied by release of vasoactive substances that continue to reduce blood supply.[15] In NQW MI there is more prolonged (up to 1 h) transient occlusion.[16] From this description it is clear that the distinction between Q and NQW MI is somewhat arbitrary.

Management

Treatment aims consist of control of symptoms and prevention of MI and death. This can be achieved by instituting anti-ischaemic and antithrombotic therapy in the first instance, and if this is not proving successful by mechanical revascularization.

Anti-ischaemic therapy

- Restriction of activity to reduce oxygen demand and administration of oxygen is appropriate in all patients, as indeed may be the use of opioids.

- Detection and correction of an obvious precipitating factor such as anaemia, fever, thyrotoxicosis, hypoxia, tachyarrhythmias, aortic stenosis or sympathomimetic drugs.

- Administration of buccal then IV nitrates is effective at relieving pain in a majority of patients. However, in patients with ongoing symptoms it must be remembered that tolerance will develop within 24–48 h unless a 'nitrate-free period' can be incorporated. As with Q-wave MI there is no convincing evidence of prognostic benefit.

- β-Blockers should be used in all patients with out contraindications, and in selected patients may be given IV. The prognostic benefits are not as clear cut as with Q-wave MI but it is likely that significant benefit is obtained.

- Calcium channel blockers are useful anti-ischaemic agents and should be used in conjunction with β-blockers or in patients where β-blockers are contraindicated. Short-acting dihydropyridines should not be used. There is some evidence to suggest that NQW MI may derive benefit from verapamil or diltiazem.[17]

- Nicorandil, as described previously, has very important anti-anginal actions and is frequently used in conjunction with other agents in this area. Recently it has been proposed that there may be further protective effects of using this agent in unstable angina.[18]

- Cholesterol lowering also has a part to play in these syndromes as there is increasing evidence that the use of statins can help stabilize the plaque over a short period.

Anti-thrombotic therapy

- Aspirin once again is the cornerstone of anti-platelet therapy, producing 50% reduction in MI and death at 3 months.[19] Newer oral anti-platelet drugs such as ticlopidine have an unfavourable safety profile; however, the closely related clopidogrel is much safer in long-term use, although its place in the management of UA remains unclear. Consideration should be given to using clopidogrel if a patient is genuinely intolerant of aspirin.

- Heparin, when used IV, reduces the incidence of recurrent ischaemia and progression to Q-wave MI.[20] Use of IV heparin requires careful monitoring of the level of anticoagulation and is relatively labour-intensive. The advent of the low molecular weight heparins has simplified the process and because of their almost complete bioavailability their action is more predictable and monitoring is not necessary. They must be given twice daily by subcutaneous injection for at least 3 days and they appear to have a similar efficacy to IV heparin. Evidence is also emerging from the recently-published Fast Revascularization during Instability in Coronary Artery Disease (FRISC) II study that longer term outpatient therapy (45 days) can produce further benefits.[21]

- Glycoprotein (GP) IIb/IIIa receptor antagonists is a group of agents with very potent anti-platelet actions. The group inhibits the final common step of platelet activation and its use has become widespread in the field of interventional cardiology to prevent acute and subacute coronary thrombosis. More information on their use in patients with UA and NQW MI suggests that there is less requirement to proceed to revascularization.[22] Pretreatment of patients who eventually do have percutaneous revascularization also lessens the risks of angioplasty.[23] Their use is currently limited by the high costs involved.

- Thrombin inhibitors have been extensively investigated in unstable angina, with varying results. Some promising new information is becoming available, but currently the use of these agents is not recommended.

Mechanical revascularization

Coronary angiography is indicated for:

- Patients with continuing uncertainty about the diagnosis of UA.

- Patients who continue to have chest pains despite medical therapy.

- Patients with ongoing chest pain and a history of previous angioplasty or coronary artery bypass surgery.

- Patients with a recent history of UA and demonstrable evidence of easily inducible ischaemia.

As with revascularization in the setting of acute Q-wave MI, revascularization in UA and NQW MI is high risk when compared with elective procedures. Activated platelets and often thrombus are present, increasing the risks of acute thrombosis especially if intracoronary stents are used. The intensive anti-platelet regimens currently used, with ticlopidine and GP IIb/IIIa inhibitors, reduce the incidence of complications. Despite this, it is debatable whether patients with these syndromes require early intervention. The VANQUISH trial[24] showed raised mortality with an invasive approach early after NQW MI. However many observational studies and the randomised TIMI IIIb[25] and FRISC II[26] trials suggest an early invasive approach is more beneficial.

Table 2 – Canadian Cardiovascular Society Classification (CCSC) of angina pectoris.

Class	Description of stage
I	Ordinary physical activity does not cause angina, such as walking or climbing stairs. Angina occurs with strenuous, rapid or prolonged exertion at work or recreation
II	Slight limitation of ordinary activity. Angina occurs on walking or climbing stairs quickly, walking uphill, walking or climbing stairs after meals, in the cold, in wind, under emotional stress, or only during the first few hours after awakening. Walking more than two blocks on the level and climbing more than one flight of ordinary stairs at normal pace under normal conditions
III	Marked limitations of ordinary physical activity. Angina occurs on walking one to two blocks on the level and climbing more than one flight of stairs in normal conditions at normal pace
IV	Inability to carry on any physical activity without discomfort: anginal symptoms may be present at rest

Further reading

The Unstable Coronary Artery Disease Council. *Managing Unstable Coronary Artery Disease. A Practical Guide*. Medical Action Communications, 1998. London

References

1. Phibbs B. 'Transmural' versus 'subendocardial' myocardial infarction: an electrocardiographic myth. *J Am Coll Cardiol* 1983; **1**: 561.

2. Boersma E, Maas ACP, Deckers JW *et al*. Early thrombolytic treatment in acute myocardial infarction: reappraisal of the golden hour. *Lancet* 1996; **348**: 771–5.

3. The GUSTO Investigators. An international randomised trial comparing four thrombolytic therapies for acute myocardial infarction. *N Engl J Med* 1993; **329**: 673–82.

4. Langer A, Goodman SG, Topol EJ *et al*. for the LATE study investigators. Late assessment of thrombolytic efficacy (LATE) study: prognosis in patients with non-Q-wave myocardial infarction. *J Am Coll Cardiol* 1996; **27**: 1327–32.

5. White HD. Thrombolytic therapy for patients with acute myocardial infarction presenting after six hours. *Lancet* 1992; **340**: 221–2.

6. Fibrinolytic Therapy Trialists' (FTT) Collaborative Group. Indications for thrombolytic therapy in suspected acute myocardial infarction: collaborative overview of early mortality and major morbidity results from all randomized trials of more than 1000 patients. *Lancet* 1994; **343**: 311–22.

7. Kennedy JW, Ritchie JL, Davis KB et al. The Western Washington randomised trial of intra coronary streptokinase in acute myocardial infarction. N Engl J Med 1985; 312: 1073–8.

8. The GUSTO Angiographic Investigators. The effects of tissue plasminogen activator, streptokinase, or both on coronary artery patency, ventricular function, and survival, after acute myocardial infarction. *N Engl J Med* 1993; **329**: 1615–22.

9. ISIS–2 (Second International Study of Infarct Survival) Collaborative Group. Randomized trial of intravenous streptokinase, oral aspirin, both, or neither among 17187 cases of suspected acute myocardial infarction. *Lancet* 1988; **2**(8607): 349–60

10. Sleight P (for the ISIS Study Group). Beta blockade early in acute myocardial infarction. *Am J Cardiol* 1987; **60**: 6A–12A.

11. Sleight P. Professor Peter Sleight's reflections on the use of β-blocking agents after myocardial infarction. *Am Heart J* 1997; **134**: S15–20.

12. Scrutinino D, Biasco MG, Rizzon P. Thrombolysis in unstable angina: results of clinical studies. *Am J Cardiol* 1991; **68**: 99B–104B.

13. Braunwald E, Jones RH, Mark DB et al. Diagnosing and managing unstable angina. *Circulation* 1994; **90**: 613–22.

14. Lindahl B, Venge P, Wallentin L for the FRISC Study Group. Relation between troponin-t and the risk of subsequent cardiac events in unstable coronary artery disease. *Circulation* 1996; **93**: 1651–7.

15. Fuster V, Badimon L, Badimon JJ, Chesbro JH. The pathogenesis of coronary artery disease and the acute coronary syndromes. *N Engl J Med* 1992; **326**: 242–50, 310–18.

16. Braunwald E, Jones RH, Mark DB et al. Diagnosing and managing unstable angina. *Circulation* 1994; **90**: 631–22.

17. Sleight P. Calcium antagonists during and after myocardial infarction. *Drugs* 1996; **51**: 216–25.

18. Mizumura T, Saito S, Kamata T et al. Effects of nicorandil on myocardial ischaemia during balloon angioplasty. *Cardiovas Drugs Ther* 1993; **7 (suppl. 2)**: 454.

19. Lewis HD, Davis JW, Archibald DG *et al.* Protective effects of aspirin against acute MI and death in men with unstable angina. Results of a Veterans' Co-operative study. *N Engl J Med* 1983; **309**: 396.

20. Oler A, Whooley MA, Oler J, Grady D. Adding heparin to aspirin reduces the incidence of myocardial infarction and death inpatients with unstable angina. A meta-analysis. *J Am Med Assoc* 1996; **276**: 881–5.

21. Wallentin L, (for the Fragmin and fast revascularisation during instability in coronary artery disease (FRISC II) investigators. Long term low molecular mass heparin in unstable coronary artery disease : FRISC II prospective ran-domised multicentre study. Lancet 1999 : 354 : 701-7.

22. Schulman SP, Goldschmidt PJ, Topol EJ *et al.* Effects of integrilin, a platelet glycoprotein IIb/IIIa receptor antagonist, in unstable angina: a randomised multi-center trial. *Circulation* 1996; **94**: 2083–9.

23. The CAPTURE Investigators. Randomized placebo controlled trial of abcix-imab before and during coronary intervention in refractory angina: the CAP-TURE study. *Lancet* 1997; **349**: 1429–34.

24. Bohen WE, O'Rourke RA, Crawford MH et al. Outcomes in patients with acute non Q wave myocardial infarction randomly assigned to an invasive as compared with conservative management strategy : Veterans affairs non Q wave infarction strategies in hospital (VANQUISH) trial investigators. N Eng J Med 1998 : 338 : 1785-92.

25. McCullough PH, O'Neil W, Graham M et al. A prospective randomised trial of triage angioplasty in acute coronary syndromes ineligible for thrombolytic therapy. J Am Coll cardiol 1998 : 32 : 596-605.

26. Wallentin L (for the FRISC II investigators). Invasive compared with nonin-vasive treatment in unstable coronary disease : FRISC II prospective ran-domised multicentre study. Lancet 1999 : 354 : 708-15.

13

CARDIOGENIC SHOCK

The incidence of cardiogenic shock is about 5–10% in patients with myocardial infarction and accounts for the most frequent cause of death in this group of patients. The in-hospital mortality rate remains high once cardiogenic shock is established and is often about 70–80%. In the majority of patients, shock occurs as a result of extensive ischaemic damage to the left ventricle secondary to acute anterior myocardial infarction and tends to occur within the first 24 h of infarction. Other potentially reversible causes of cardiogenic shock need to be excluded and tend to occur after the first 24 h. These include patients developing shock following right ventricular infarction or as a consequence of mechanical complications such as ventricular septal rupture, papillary muscle infarction leading to severe mitral regurgitation and cardiac tamponade due to haemorrhagic pericardial effusion. The incidence of cardiogenic shock is higher in old age,[1,2] females,[3] history of previous myocardial infarction[1] and patients with diabetes mellitus or hyperglycaemia on admission.

DIAGNOSIS OF CARDIOGENIC SHOCK

There are various definitions of cardiogenic shock but the condition is characterized by:

- Persistent systemic hypotension (BP < 90 mmHg).

- Clammy extremities.

- End organ hypoperfusion.

- Confusion.

- Oliguria (< 30 ml/h).

- Cardiac index (CI) < 1.8 l/min/m^2.

- Elevated ventricular filling pressures.

- Crepitations on auscultation.

- Radiological evidence of pulmonary oedema.

- High pulmonary capillary wedge pressure (PCWP).

As soon as cardiogenic shock is suspected it may be necessary to insert a right heart catheter to measure PCWP and cardiac output. The correct management of cardiogenic shock depends on its aetiology and this can be determined by interpretation of the right heart pressures, right heart oxygen saturations and the results of either transthoracic (TTE) or transoesophageal echocardiography (TOE).

MANAGEMENT OF CARDIOGENIC SHOCK DUE TO SEVERE LEFT VENTRICULAR DYSFUNCTION

General measures

- Correct metabolic conditions that arise secondary to poor LV function, e.g. hypoxemia and acidosis.

- Treat incidental arrhythmias.

- Correct hyperglycaemia.

- Adequate pain relief.

- Ensure that hypotension is not secondary to either poor fluid intake or excessive fluid loss due to over enthusiastic use of diuretic therapy.

Medical support

Patients with cardiogenic shock are initially treated with inotropes in an attempt to stabilize their haemodynamic state. IV dobutamine (5–20 mcg/kg/min) is frequently used to produce an improvement in cardiac output and dopamine (2.5 mcg/kg/min) to improve renal perfusion. The use of IV nitrate to reduce afterload although desirable is often limited by systemic hypotension. Reversing systemic hypotension with noradrenaline can lead to an improvement in myocardial perfusion and oxygenation but does not appear to alter mortality rate if used as a stand alone treatment.

Mechanical support

Intra-aortic balloon pump (IABP) (see also Chapter 9)

IABP insertion is relatively simple to perform and can be performed in ITU or CCU without the aid of radiological screening. It can of course be inserted under direct X-ray screening if available. The balloon is inserted via the femoral artery with or without a femoral sheath under local anaesthetic. Inflation and deflation of the balloon synchronized with the cardiac cycle results in augmentation of coronary blood flow as well as producing a reduction of afterload and impedance.[4] This has the effect of increasing the cardiac index (CI) and diastolic pressure. Non-randomized trial data from the prethrombolytic era revealed that if patients with cardiogenic shock refractory to medical therapy were placed on an IABP a high percentage of patients initially improved and could be stabilized. However, the in-hospital mortality rate was still about 80%. It is clear that for patients in cardiogenic shock secondary to myocardial infarction IABP as a stand-alone treatment does not improve outcome unless it is used in conjunction with some form of coronary reperfusion.

Coronary reperfusion and revascularization

There is little information that specifically examines thrombolysis in the context of cardiogenic shock.

- The GISSI trial[5] randomized 11 806 patients to receive IV streptokinase or placebo, 281 patients presented in cardiogenic shock. The mortality rate in the thrombolysed group was not significantly different from the placebo group (69.9 versus 70.1% respectively).

- The ISIS–3 trial[6] compared three thrombolytic agents, streptokinase, tissue plasminogen activator (t-PA) and anisoylated plasminogen activator complex (APSAC). The rates of cardiogenic shock development were similar.

- The GUSTO trial[7] reported a lower incidence of cardiogenic shock in patients treated with 'front loaded' t-PA compared with streptokinase (5.1 versus 6.6%).

It may well be that rapid and successful coronary reperfusion can influence the outcome of patients presenting in cardiogenic shock and the condition should not be regarded as a contraindication to thrombolysis.

Percutaneous transluminal coronary angioplasty (PTCA) and coronary artery bypass surgery (CABG)

There is a considerable amount of retrospective data addressing PTCA in the setting of cardiogenic shock. The Duke series[8] was a non-randomized trial involving 200 patients with cardiogenic shock post-myocardial infarction. Coronary angiography was performed on 154 patients. Patients with a closed infarct-related artery (IRA) were treated medically, underwent CABG or PTCA. Those who underwent successful PTCA had an in hospital survival rate of 55%. Bias influenced these results since clinicians can identify those patients who may do well and refer early for investigation and revascularization, and patients with a grim outlook may not be referred or die before being investigated. The prospective SHOCK registry[9] examined the data on 251 patients with cardiogenic shock from 1992 to 1993. The in-hospital mortality rate was 70%. No parameter that predicted survival in patients undergoing early revascularization was discovered, including age, sex, thrombolysis, time from infarct to shock and time from onset of shock to revascularization.

Little data are available about the benefit of CABG in cardiogenic shock post-myocardial infarction. What there is is non-randomized and consists of small patient numbers. The in-hospital mortality rate is in the range 40–80%.

Summary

- Once cardiogenic shock due to myocardial infarction is suspected, prompt diagnosis and initiation of treatment is essential if survival is to be improved.

- Support medically in the first instance.

- Liaise with the cardiologist about invasive treatment including IABP insertion and potential coronary angiography and PTCA.

SHOCK SECONDARY TO RIGHT VENTRICULAR INFARCTION

A significant inferior or posterior myocardial infarct can result in right ventricular dysfunction and shock. The prognosis if diagnosed and treated promptly is considerably better than shock associated with left ventricular dysfunction. The mortality rate is about 20%.

- Patients with RV infarction are usually hypotensive, have a raised jugular venous pressure and no pulmonary congestion (a clear chest on auscultation).

- The diagnosis of RV infarct can be confirmed by performing a right-sided chest lead on the ECG (V4R). ST elevation in this lead is diagnostic. It has to be remembered that this feature may be transient and its absence does not rule out RV infarct.

- The insertion of a right heart catheter can aid the diagnosis and the typical findings are a low or normal PCWP and an elevated CVP. The treatment consists of rapid infusion of fluid to maintain the PCWP at about 15 mmHg. Despite adequate fluid replacement some patients remain hypotensive and may require support with dobutamine or dopamine. Should heart block develop, dual chamber pacing is more appropriate than single-chamber pacing since AV synchrony is maintained.

MECHANICAL CAUSES OF CARDIOGENIC SHOCK (SEE ALSO CHAPTERS 8 AND 17)

A subgroup of patients that develop cardiac failure and shock post-myocardial infarction do so as a result of mechanical complications, namely ventricular septal rupture (VSD), mitral regurgitation and left ventricular free wall rupture. Aggressive support and surgical intervention can improve the outlook of selected patients.

Ventricular septal defect

Septal rupture is not common, having an incidence rate of 1–2%.[9] Rupture is most likely to occur within the first week post-infarction. More recently it has been suggested that the interval from infarction to rupture is shorter in patients who had received thrombolytic therapy and can develop at about 24 h post-infarct. Men seem to be affected more often than women, and in the majority of cases the rupture complicates the patients' first myocardial infarct. The majority of ruptures are secondary to anterior myocardial infarction, which results in an anterior or apical defect. Inferior infarction produces a defect in the inferior septum.

- Patients develop a new loud systolic murmur heard best at the left sternal edge in association with a deterioration in their clinical condition leading to cardiac failure and cardiogenic shock. Some patients may also experience a recurrence of ischaemic pain.

- The diagnosis of ventricular septal rupture can be confirmed by echocardiography (see Chapter 8, figure 1) and right heart catheterization. Both techniques can be performed at the bedside, are quick and, in the case of right heart catheter, relatively safe. With a right heart catheter in place, the oxygen saturation in the right atrium and pulmonary artery can be determined to confirm the diagnosis and the pulmonary to systemic flow ratio can be calculated.

The outlook for patients who are not surgically treated is grim. The majority (about 90%) dies within 2 weeks if not corrected. As soon as the diagnosis is confirmed, management should be directed at stabilizing the patient haemodynamically with a view to surgical intervention. Discussions between the cardiologist and the cardiac surgeon at this time are essential. IABP support reduces LV afterload and increases systemic cardiac output. This device should be used in conjunction with inotropic support to maintain renal function and blood pressure. Coronary angiography is usually required pre-operatively. However, coronary bypass and defect repair has been a controversial point.

The in-hospital survival rate of patients undergoing multiple grafts and repair may not be different to those undergoing repair only, but the long-term outcome is improved. More controversy exists about the timing of surgery. Initially repair was only attempted in patients who had survived for a few months post-infarct.

Later surgeons performed the repair in the acute phase especially in patients who deteriorated haemodynamically soon after their infarct and septal rupture. With an early surgical approach, a 25% hospital mortality rate can be expected; the operative mortality rate is about 10%. Experienced centres in the USA report 5- and 10-year survival rates of 73 and 48% respectively in patients undergoing two- and three-vessel bypass surgery.

Summary

- If you do not suspect it you will never diagnose it!
- Onset of new harsh systolic murmur.
- Development of left ventricular failure and shock.
- Organize urgent echocardiography.
- Consider right heart catheter.
- Contact the cardiology team **EARLY**.
- Initial treatment consists of IABP insertion and medical support.
- Coronary angiography.
- Cardiac surgery, repair of defect with or without bypass surgery.

Mitral incompetence (see also Chapter 17)

Papillary muscle rupture complicating myocardial infarction occurs at between 0.5 and 5%.[10] With complete rupture of the papillary muscle the 24-h survival rate is 25%. If the rupture is only partial, survival is considerably better, with a 24 h survival rate of > 70% and 50% at 1 month.

- Acute papillary rupture typically presents with severe congestive cardiac failure 3–10 days following myocardial infarction. Whereas a septal rupture complicates a large infarct, papillary rupture often complicates smaller infarcts. The patient's clinical situation deteriorates rapidly because the left atrium and LV have not had time to adapt to the mitral regurgitation. Despite good left ventricular function, the left atrial pressure increases resulting in pulmonary oedema. Cardiogenic shock develops as a result of increased workload and a dilated, overloaded left ventricle.

Acute mitral regurgitation should be suspected in patients who develop shortness of breath, shock and a new apical systolic murmur. Ventricular septal rupture has a similar presentation.

Echocardiography (see Chapter 8), which can be performed at the patients bedside, is the best test to confirm the diagnosis and right heart catheterization reveals tall 'V' waves in the PCWP traces and pulmonary hypertension.

The initial treatment consists of IABP and inotropic support. If the patient is stable, coronary angiography should be considered before surgery. Mitral valve replacement is usually required in patients who have suffered complete papillary rupture.

Summary

- If you do not suspect it you will never diagnose it!

- Development of cardiogenic shock.

- New apical systolic murmur.

- Organize echocardiography.

- Right heart catheter.

- Contact the cardiology team **EARLY**.

- IABP and inotropic support.

- Coronary angiography depending on situation.

- Cardiac surgery.

Left ventricular rupture

This condition tends to be fatal in the majority of cases and often the patient dies before any diagnostic tests can be performed. Rupture usually arises in an area of fresh infarction at about 3–6 days post-infarct. The condition appears to affect women more than men, and is more frequent in older patients. Patients who develop cardiac rupture have chest pain and signs of cardiac tamponade. A patient may therefore be progressing well post-infarct and suddenly become haemodynamically very unstable.

- Echocardiography at the bedside is helpful in diagnosing a new or increasing pericardial effusion and tamponade.

- Pericardiocentesis should be performed. It may stabilize the patient and in some the rupture may heal. However, surgery should be considered as soon as the diagnosis is made.

Summary

- Cardiac rupture has an incidence of about 5%.

- Patients rapidly deteriorate with signs of cardiac tamponade.

- Echocardiography is a useful diagnostic tool.

- Pericardiocentesis may be life saving.

- Immediate cardiac surgery should be considered since the outlook is grim.

Further reading

Califf RM, Bengtson JR. Cardiogenic shock. *N Engl J Med* 1994; **330**: 1724–30.

Webb JG. Interventional management of cardiogenic shock. *Can J Cardiol* 1998; **14**: 233–44.

References

1. Goldberg RJ, Gore JM, Alpert JS *et al.* Cardiogenic shock after acute myocardial infarction. Incidence and mortality from a community wise perspective, 1975 to 1988. *N Engl J Med*; **325**: 1117–22. Year?

2. Hands ME, Rutherford JD, Muller JE *et al.* The in hospital development of cardiogenic shock after myocardial infarction: Incidence, predictors of occurrence, outcome and prognostic factors. *J Am Coll Cardiol* 1989; **14**: 40–6.

3. Holmes DR, Bates E for the GUSTO Investigators. Cardiogenic shock during myocardial infarction. The GUSTO experience with thrombolytic therapy. *Circulation* 1993; **88**: I–25 (abstr).

4. Fuchs RM, Brin KD, Brinker JA *et al.* Augmentation of regional coronary blood flow by intra-aortic balloon counterpulsation in patients with unstable angina. *Circulation* 1983; **68**: 117–23.

5. Gruppo Italiano per lo Studio della Streptokinase nell'Infarcto Micardio (GISSI). Effectiveness of intravenous thrombolytic treatment in acute myocardial infarction. *Lancet* 1986; **i**: 397–401.

6. ISSIS–3. Third International Study of Infarct Survival Collaborative Group. A randomized comparison of streptokinase vs tissue plasminogen activator vs anistreplase and of aspirin plus heparin vs aspirin alone among 41,299 cases of suspected acute myocardial infarction. *Lancet*; 339: 753–70. 1992

7. The GUSTO Investigators. An International randomized trial comparing four thrombolytic strategies for acute myocardial infarction. *N Engl J Med* 1993; **329**: 673–82.

8. Benggston JR, Kaplin AJ, Pieper KS *et al.* Prognosis in cardiogenic shock after myocardial infarction in the intervention era. *J Am Coll Cardiol* 1992; **20**: 1482–9.

9. Hutchins G. Rupture of the interventricular septum in myocardial infarction. *Am Heart J* 1979; **97**: 165.

10. Chawa E, Gonzalez A, Bahr RD *et al*. Papillary muscle rupture: a reversible cause of cardiogenic shock. *Md Med J* 1992; **41**: 893–7.

14

HEART FAILURE

- Heart failure is a complex syndrome but essentially it occurs when a cardiac abnormality results in the cardiac output failing to meet the requirements of the body's metabolism.

- It is a common condition and an important cause of morbidity and mortality, having a significant impact on health service resources.

- Patients with a minor degree of cardiac impairment may be asymptomatic but as compensatory mechanisms, i.e. neurohormonal activation, ventricular dilation and hypertrophy, fail they may present acutely or more insidiously with a more chronic picture.

ACUTE LEFT VENTRICULAR FAILURE (LVF)

This condition is a life-threatening medical emergency and should always be regarded as such. The commonest cause for this is myocardial infarction, but it has to be remembered that there are other causes of acute LVF that include chronic hypertensive heart disease, acute mitral regurgitation, acute aortic regurgitation, myocarditis and mitral stenosis. Rarer causes include thyrotoxicosis, Beri Beri and Paget's disease.

Pulmonary oedema may develop, resulting in a patient typically becoming acutely dyspnoeic, coughing and producing a pink, frothy liquid. Patients are often sweaty, cyanosed and restless.

It is worth noting that pulmonary oedema can arise in the absence of a failing LV (table 1).

- Auscultation of the heart may prove difficult but a third heart sound is present with or without a sinus tachycardia.

- The lungs are moist, initially with basal crackles that extend towards the apices as the condition worsens. The crackles are not affected by coughing.

Table 1 –Causes of pulmonary oedema in the absence of a failing LV.

- Cardiac causes with normal LV—mitral stenosis, cardiac tamponade, cardiac arrhytmia

- ARDS

- Lymphatic insufficiency—lymphangitis carcinomatosis, fibrosing lymphangitis

- Other causes—high altitude pulmonary oedema, neurogenic pulmonary oedema, heroin overdose, post-cardioversion, eclampsia, post-cardiopulmonary bypass

Investigations

Acute left ventricular failure can often be diagnosed on clinical grounds but a complete diagnosis requires a cause for the LVF.

ECG

May be abnormal and reveals ST elevation suggesting an acute myocardial infarction, ST depression in unstable angina, bundle branch block or a tachyarrhythmia. The presence of left ventricular hypertrophy may indicate underlying aortic valve disease or hypertension.

Chest X-ray

The chest X-ray shows Kerley B lines due to interstitial oedema and a diffuse haziness as a result of alveolar fluid. Dilation of the upper lobe veins is also seen.

Blood tests

Routine blood tests should include cardiac enzymes, electrolytes and a full blood count. Other investigations such as transthoracic echo and central monitoring can be deferred until emergency treatment and stabilization of the patient has been achieved.

Initial treatment of acute pulmonary oedema

- The patient should be in a sitting position. Most patients will have already recognized that they feel much worse lying flat or semi-recumbent.

- High concentration oxygen should be given. Caution should be taken if there is a suspicion of co-existing chronic airways disease. Repeat arterial blood gas analysis may be required.

- Diamorphine by slow IV injection. This has several effects: it diminishes both patient distress and central sympathetic outflow, which causes venous and arteriolar constriction. In the setting of pulmonary oedema this results in venous dilation. An anti-emetic should be given with diamorphine. Avoid giving IM injections because if the patient has had a myocardial infarction then thrombolysis may cause significant haematoma formation. Also if primary angioplasty were to be performed, the heparin or platelet antagonists used in the procedure could also result in significant IM bleeding.

- IV diuretics such as frusemide 50–100 mg or bumetanide 1–2 mg. The effect of IV diuretics is immediate, which suggests that the initial effects are not on the kidney but on venodilation. There is a more delayed diuretic response.

- Venous vasodilators – patients with acute pulmonary oedema often have an elevation of arterial and left ventricular end-diastolic pressure, depression of cardiac output and elevation of systemic vascular resistance. Vasodilator therapy reduces systemic and pulmonary vascular pressures. An infusion of glycerine trinitrate or isosorbide dinitrate reduces preload and is frequently used. Hypotension is common and infusions of these agents should be commenced only if the systolic blood pressure is > 100 mmHg. If possible, patients should have invasive arterial monitoring. The infusion rates should be increased to the maximum dose that is tolerated in severe cases.

- Treat any aggravating arrhythmia appropriately and at the other end of the spectrum if pulmonary oedema occurs in a patient with significant bradycardia, e.g. in the setting of acute myocardial infarction insert a temporary pacing wire to restore the heart rate to an appropriate rate.

- Mechanical ventilation – whatever the cause of pulmonary oedema, repeated arterial blood gas analysis is important. If significant hypoxia without hypercapnia develops despite adequate inhalation of oxygen, assisted ventilation may be considered. This subject is further explored in Chapter 4.

DIASTOLIC DYSFUNCTION IN HEART FAILURE

Abnormalities of diastolic filling may be the main problem in some patients with heart failure. Failure of the ventricle to relax (reduced compliance) occurs with reduced systolic function in heart failure. However, some patients present with pure diastolic failure with elevated filling pressures with normal systolic function as measured by LVEF. The non-compliant ventricle may lead to markedly elevated cardiac filling pressures that can precipitate pulmonary oedema. Calcium antagonists have been used by some clinicians when this problem is suspected. In acute heart failure with diastolic dysfunction, inotropes that relax the ventricle (positive lusitropic agents) such as Enoximone may be useful.

CHRONIC HEART FAILURE

Pharmacological therapy

Diuretics

For symptomatic treatment of fluid overload that produces clinical symptoms of peripheral oedema and pulmonary congestion, diuretics are essential. If possible, diuretics should be prescribed in combination with an angiotensin-converting enzyme (ACE) inhibitor. Mild failure can often be treated with a thiazide diuretic, but it becomes less effective as the glomerular filtration rate falls, a situation commonly found in elderly patients with heart failure. In the setting of severe heart failure, thiazide diuretics have a synergistic effect with loop diuretics and can be used in combination. This combination is more efficient than simply increasing the dose of loop diuretic. Metolazone is usually added as a 'drug of last resort' to loop diuretics.

Potassium-sparing diuretics

The majority of patients with heart failure who are receiving diuretics will also be on an ACE inhibitor. In general terms, potassium-sparing diuretics should not be used in combination with ACE inhibitors. If there is a persisting hypokalaemia with or without ACE inhibitors, a potassium-sparing diuretic can be used either to prevent or treat diuretic-induced hypokalaemia. If a potassium-sparing diuretic is being used, the serum creatinine and potassium should be measured weekly during initiation and until the values remain stable. Once stable, measurements should be performed at 3–6-monthly intervals.

ACE inhibitors

These drugs are indicated in all stages of symptomatic heart failure secondary to systolic cardiac dysfunction. All patients being treated with a diuretic for heart failure should be considered for treatment with an ACE inhibitor.

- In patients with asymptomatic left ventricular dysfunction, prescribing an ACE inhibitor reduces the development of heart failure and in-patient hospital episodes related to heart failure. However, there is no significant difference in mortality rate.[1]

- In patients with symptomatic heart failure, ACE inhibitors improve symptoms, reduce hospitalization and reduce the mortality rate.[2,3]

- Complications of ACE therapy include hypotension, syncope, deterioration of renal function and hyperkalaemia. A dry irritating cough may result in ACE withdrawal in about 15–20% of patients, but a history of a previous ACE-induced cough is only a relative contraindication to prescribing an ACE inhibitor.

Absolute contraindications for initiating ACE inhibitor therapy:

- bilateral renal artery stenosis
- angioedema during previous therapy
- serum potassium > 5.5 mmol/l.[1]

Senior advice should be sought in the following patients:

- heart failure of unknown aetiology
- systolic BP < 100 mmHg
- renal impairment
- severe heart failure
- underlying valve disease

Cardiac glycosides

The specific indications for the use of digoxin are when a fast ventricular rate in atrial fibrillation is present in any degree of heart failure secondary to systolic dysfunction. In asymptomatic patients with dysfunction and atrial fibrillation, digoxin can be used for rate control. The role of digoxin in combination with diuretics and ACE inhibitors in patients with NYHA Class III and IV failure due to systolic dysfunction who are in sinus rhythm is debatable. There may be a symptomatic benefit and less admissions due to worsening failure, but there is no mortality rate benefit in patients with NYHA Class II–IV in sinus rhythm.

β-Blockers and heart failure

The CIBIS-II (Cardiac Insufficency Bisoprolol Study II)[4] was stopped early because of the significant mortality benefit in those patients receiving Bisoprolol. The trial was a double blind trial enrolling 2647 symptomatic patients with NYHA class III or IV failure with LV ejection fraction of 35% or less receiving standard therapy with diuretics and ACE inhibitors. Patients were assigned to Bisoprolol 1.25mg (n=1327) increasing to 10mg per day if tolerated or placebo (n=1320). All cause mortality was lower with Bisoprolol (11.8% vs 17.3% deaths). However, there is no data currently to support the use in patients with severe class IV symptoms or recent instability.

Carvedilol combines non-selective β-blockade with weak α-blockade and antioxidant properties. Clinical trials with carvedilol in heart failure have been performed.

- In a US clinical trial, 696 patients received carvedilol and 398 a placebo in addition to ACE inhibitor therapy. There was a 65% reduction in all-cause mortality rate and a 27% reduction in hospitalization for cardiovascular events in patients receiving carvedilol.[5]

- In a smaller study of 415 patients with ischaemic cardiac failure (NYHA Class I–IV), carvedilol or placebo was added to ACE inhibitors, diuretics and digitalis. There was 26% reduction in the combined end point, mortality rate and hospitalization with carvedilol.[6]

The mechanism behind the beneficial effect of β-blockers in heart failure is uncertain. The slowed heart rate may result in improved diastolic ventricular function enhancing systolic function. Alternatively β-receptor down-regulation in chronic heart failure may be reversed by a low dose of β-blockers.

Vasodilators

The combination of hydralazine and isosorbide dinitrate can be used when ACE inhibitors can not be used for reasons of intolerance or if contraindicated. The doses of hydralazine, up to 300 mg/day and isosorbide dinitrate 160 mg/day in the presence of diuretics and cardiac glycosides, possibly have some effect on mortality rate, but not on the rates of hospitalization. The effects of these agents either in combination or alone when added to an ACE inhibitor are not known. Likewise, there is no evidence to support the use of either of these agents alone. Development of tolerance to nitrates occurs with frequent doses but can be reduced with dose intervals of 8–12 h.

Spironolactone

The effects of spironolactone on mortality and morbidity in patients with severe heart failure have now been published[7]. These patients were already receiving loop diuretics, ACE inhibitors and, in many cases, digoxin. 1663 patients were enrolled into the trial which was discontinued early after a mean follow up period of 24 months. There was a 30% reduction in the risk of death in the spironolactone group (25mg daily) compared with the placebo group. This was attributed to a lower risk of heart failure progression and sudden cardiac death. The rates of hospitalisation for worsening heart failure were also significantly lower in the spironolactone group.

Dopaminergic drugs

Currently the only orally acting dopaminergic drug available for clinical use (in some European countries) is ibopamide. A recent mortality trial was stopped prematurely due to an excess of deaths in patients with severe heart failure.[8]

There are no data to suggest the clinical use of ibopamide.

Anti-arrhythmic therapy (see also Chapters 2 and 15)

Indications for this type of treatment include atrial fibrillation and non-sustained or sustained ventricular tachycardia. Amiodarone (a class III anti-arrhythmic) has several advantages in that it is effective in the treatment of supraventricular and ventricular arrhythmias and has no significant negative inotropic effect. Class I anti-arrhythmic agents should be avoided if possible because they have pro-arrhythmic effects and are negatively inotropic.

Cardiac surgery

In patients with heart failure secondary to ischaemia, there is a possibility that chronically hypoperfused myocytes may be viable although they appear hypokinetic and akinetic. This dysfunction is the so-called hibernating myocardium. As a result of this, revascularization of heart failure patients is gaining interest.

Heart transplantation

Transplantation in end-stage heart failure patients increases survival rate, quality of life and increases exercise capacity. Recent results suggest a 5-year survival rate of 70–80%.[9] The limitations are rejection of the graft and problems associated with immunosupression, i.e. infection, renal failure, hypertension and accelerated progression of atherosclerotic disease. Contraindications for transplantation are shown in table 2.

Cardiomyoplasty

This method of treatment has been used in a very small number of patients with severe chronic heart failure. Patients initially undergoing this procedure had contraindications to transplantation or were in a poor condition generally. Patients selected for this procedure must be thought able to survive the 3-month period between isolation of the latissimus dorsi muscle and the final functioning of the muscle. Controlled studies and long-term follow-up are needed.

Table 2 –Contradictions to cardiac transplantation.

• Age > 60 years does vary from centre to centre
• Present alcohol and drug abuse
• Chronic mental disease not properly controlled
• Treated cancer with remission and < 5-year follow-up
• Systemic disease with multi-organ involvement
• Uncontrolled hypertension
• Severe renal failure
• Fixed high pulmonary vascular resistance
• Recent thrombo-embolic complications
• Significant liver impairment

Ventricular assist devices and artificial hearts

There are several assist devices undergoing evaluation and like the artificial heart they tend to be used as a bridge to transplantation.

Further reading

Konstam MA, Remme WJ. Treatment guidelines in heart failure. *Prog Cardiovasc Dis* 1998; **48**: 65–72.

Stevenson LW, Massie BM, Francis GS. Optimizing therapy for complex or refractory heart failure: a management algorithm. *Am Heart J* 1998; **135**: S293–309.

References

1. The SOLVD Investigators. Effects of enalapril on mortality and the development of heart failure in asymptomatic patients with reduced left ventricular ejection fractions. *N Engl J Med* 1992; **327**: 685–91.

2. CONSENSUS Trial Study Group. Effects of enalapril on mortality in severe congestive heart failure. Results of the north Scandinavian enalapril survival study. *N Engl J Med* 1987; **316**: 1429–35.

3. The SOLVD Investigators. Effects of enalapril on survival in patients with reduced left ventricular ejection fractions and congestive heart failure. *N Engl J Med* 1992; **325**: 293–302.

4. CIBIS-II investigators and committees. The Cardiac Insufficency Bisoprolol Study II (CIBIS-II): a randomised trial. *Lancet* 1999 ; 353 : 9-13.

5. Packer M, Birstow MR, Cohn J et al. and the US Heart Failure Study Group. The effect of carvedilol on morbidity and mortality in patients with chronic heart failure. *N Engl J Med* 1996; **334**: 1349–55.

6. Australian/New Zealand Heart Failure Collaborative Group. Randomized placebo-controlled trial of carvedilol in patients with congestive heart failure due to ischaemic heart disease. *Lancet* 1996; **349**: 375–80.

7. Zannad PB, Remme WJ, Cody R et al. The effect of spironolactone on morbidity and mortality in patients with severe heart failure. *N Eng J Med* 1999; **341**: 709–17.

8. Mededeling van het College ter beoordeling van geneesmiddelen betreffende ibopamide (inopamil). *Ned Tijdschr Geneeskd* 1996; **139**: 2059.

9. The Registry of the International Society for Heart and Lung Transplantation. Ninth Official Report 1992. *J Heart Lung Transplant* 1992; **11**: 599–606.

15

ACUTE MANAGEMENT OF CARDIAC ARRHYTHMIAS

GENERAL STRATEGY

- Single rhythm strip or cardiac monitor may be inadequate for diagnosis.
- Twelve-lead ECG is often essential for diagnosis.
- Atrial activity is often the key to diagnosis (best seen in leads II and V_1).
- Always keep a hard copy of the arrhythmia (either rhythm strip or 12-lead ECG) that is of diagnostic or therapeutic importance. This may be important to the long-term management of the patient and particularly for pacemaker implantation.

Treatment depends on the underlying arrhythmia and will be discussed in detail below. In general, however, attention should be directed towards the underlying precipitating cause with correction of ischaemia, hypoxia, acid–base disturbance and electrolyte abnormalities. Also, many drugs will be arrhythmogenic, particularly drugs used for inotropic support.

SINUS RHYTHM

The sinus node initiates electrical activity leading to activation of atrial and ventricular myocardium during each heart beat. The sinus node lies at the junction of the superior vena cava and right atrium. As atrial activation spreads from the sinus node in an inferior direction, the P wave is upright in leads II, III and aVF, which are orientated towards the inferior surface of the heart. The atrioventricular node delays the transmission of the impulse from atria to ventricles, which is reflected by the PR interval. This is measured from the onset of the P wave to the onset of the ventricular complex. The normal PR interval ranges from 120 to 200 ms.

SINUS BRADYCARDIA

A sinus rate < 60/min as defined as sinus bradycardia. This may be physiological or caused by ischaemia, sick sinus syndrome or anti-arrhythmic drugs. It is important to exclude non-cardiac disorders such as raised intracranial pressure, and hypothyroidism and hypothermia.

Treatment is only indicated if the bradycardia is causing symptoms, haemodynamic disturbance or giving rise to tachyarrhythmia.

Treatment

- Treatment of the underlying condition.

- Temporary increase in heart rate can be achieved by atropine IV. Temporary pacing is the most effective way to increase the heart rate while the underlying condition is being rectified. Atrial pacing is preferable to ventricular pacing as the cardiac output is optimized due to preservation of atrial systole.

SINUS TACHYCARDIA

A sinus rate > 100 beats/min is defined as sinus tachycardia. Exercise or anxiety and any condition increasing sympathetic activity commonly cause sinus tachycardia.

- Sinus tachycardia is a physiological response and does not require specific treatment.

- If sinus tachycardia is excessive, treatment should be directed at the underlying condition.

- For inappropriate sinus tachycardia causing impairment in haemodynamics,[1] β-blockers are sometimes appropriate. Esmolol as an IV infusion is useful as its half-life is short when withdrawn.

- Rarely sinus tachycardia can be produced by a primary disorder of sinus node called sinus node re-entrant tachycardia.

- It is important not to be confused with either atrial flutter or atrial tachycardia with a 2:1 AV block leading to a heart rate of between 140 and 160 beats/min. The diagnosis of atrial flutter is usually made on a careful inspection of a 12-lead ECG. If diagnosis is difficult, IV adenosine can be given to cause transient AV block, which will reveal the typical 'saw tooth' atrial flutter waves.

SUPRAVENTRICULAR TACHYCARDIA

Supraventricular tachycardia is a general term for all arrhythmias originating from the atria or AV junction. They usually result in narrow ventricular complexes but have different mechanisms (table 1).

Table 1 – Mechanisms of supraventricular tachycardias.

	Re-entry	Delayed after depolarization	Abnormal automaticity
Atrial tachycardia			
Paroxysmal	+	+	
Incessant or permanent			+
Atrial flutter	+		
Atrial fibrillation	+ (multicirc)		
AV nodal tachycardia			
Common form (slow–fast)	+		
Uncommon form (fast–slow)	+		
AV junctional accelerated rhythm			
Digitalis induced		?	
Post-cardiac surgery			+
Infections			+
Ischaemic			+
AV junctional circus movement			
Paroxysmal	+		
Non-paroxysmal	+		

ATRIOVENTRICULAR NODAL RE-ENTRANT TACHYCARDIA (AVNRT)

AVNRT is probably the most common cause of paroxysmal regular supraventricular tachycardia. It is due to a re-entrant mechanism with at least two functionally distinct conduction pathways in the AV node. Rapid conduction and a long refractory period (fast pathway) characterize one pathway. The second has slow conduction velocity and a short refractory period (slow pathway). During sinus rhythm conduction is through the AV node via the fast pathway. The AVNRT is initiated by an atrial premature depolarization that blocks the fast pathway anterogradely. This can enable an impulse to propagate retrogradely over the fast pathway back to the atrium completing a re-entrant circuit.

ECG characteristics

- Negative P waves leads II, III and aVF (rarely visible due to superimposition on QRS complex).

- Regular narrow QRS complexes.

- 10% of patients will have anterograde conduction in the fast pathway and retrograde conduction in the slow pathway giving clearly visible P waves that are inverted on surface ECG leads II, III and aVF (RP interval > PR interval).

AV RE-ENTRANT TACHYCARDIA (AVRT)

- The term 're-entry' refers to re-entrant circuits involving an anomalous conduction pathway between the atria and ventricles separate from the AV node. In the Wolff–Parkinson–White syndrome (WPW) anterograde accessory pathway conduction during sinus rhythm allows ventricular pre-excitation resulting in a combination of short PR interval and d (delta) wave.

- 25% of accessory pathways are capable of only retrograde conduction and are called concealed bypass tracts as their presence is not evident on the surface ECG during sinus rhythm.

- The most common SVT in patients in WPW is AVRT.

- Tachycardia is usually initiated with a spontaneous atrial ventricular premature depolarization with retrograde conduction over the accessory pathway to the atrium.

- ECG characteristics consist of a regular narrow complex tachycardia with inverted P waves after the QRS complex (RP <PR).

- Atrial fibrillation and atrial flutter are frequently seen in patients with WPW, which can be particularly hazardous because of the properties of the accessory pathway. These patients can achieve ventricular rates that approach 300 beats/min during atrial fibrillation or atrial flutter, which can lead to ventricular fibrillation.

Treatment

- Symptoms associated with SVT can be subtle. Patients may have palpitations, light-headedness, dyspnoea, vague chest discomfort or occasionally angina. These symptoms are often more common in patients with underlying heart disease. Major complications are uncommon.

- Initial therapy can be with vagal manoeuvres such as carotid sinus massage or the Valsalva manoeuvre. This can also increase the diagnostic accuracy.

- If vagal manoeuvres do not terminate the attack, adenosine is the drug of first choice when given rapidly IV.[2]

- Of SVT, 90% is due to AV nodal re-entry or atrioventricular re-entry, terminated by 12 mg adenosine.

Care should be taken in some circumstances:

- dipyridamole potentiates the effects of adenosine

- heart transplant recipients have a denervation supersensitivity to adenosine

- patients with asthma and bronchospasm could be triggered by IV adenosine, which is a theoretical risk though rarely, if ever, seen clinically

- The calcium channel blocker verapamil, 5 mg IV, is as effective in terminating an attack. Disadvantages are hypotension. Verapamil also has a longer duration of action.

Pharmacological therapy is given in table 2. In general, polypharmacy should be avoided and, if two drugs are ineffective, particularly in a collapsed patient, electrical cardioversion should be used.

Long-term prophylactic treatment is beyond the scope of this chapter, but useful pharmacological therapy includes the use of flecainide, β-blockers including sotalol, and propafenone. However, catheter ablation using radiofrequency energy is now the first choice therapy.

Table 2 – Parenteral antiarrythmic treatment.

Drug	Dose	Common side-effects
AV node-blocking drugs		
Adenosine	6–12 mg bolus	dyspnoea, flushing, chest pain
Verapamil	0.15 mg/kg over 2 min	hypotension, bradycardia
Diltiazem	0.25–0.35 mg/kg over 2 min	hypotension, bradycardia
Digoxin	0.5–1 mg over 2–10 min	digoxin toxicity
Propranolol	1–3 mg at 1 mg/min	hypotension, bradycardia
Esmolol	50–200 mcg/kg/min IV infusion	hypotension, bradycardia
Class I anti-arrhythmic drugs		
Flecainide	2 mg/kg at 10 mg/min	hypotension
Procainamide	10–15 mg/kg at 50 mg/min	bradycardia, dizziness
Disopyramide	1–2 mg/kg over 15 min	hypotension
Quinidine	6–10 mg/kg at 10 mg/min	hypotension
Propafenone	1–2 mg/kg over 15 min	bradycardia
Class III anti-arrhythmic drugs		
Sotalol	1–1.5 mg/kg at 10 mg/min	hypotension, pro-arrhytmia
Amiodarone	5 mg/kg over 5–10 min	hypotension, bradycardia

ATRIAL FIBRILLATION

This is one of the most common cardiac arrhythmia affecting at least 10% of the > 75-year-old population. It is usually associated with either cardiac or non-cardiac disease processes. Common causes are:

- Ischaemic heart disease.
- Hypertension.
- Hyperthyroidism.
- Alcohol (acute or chronic).
- Rheumatic heart disease.
- Heart muscle disease.
- Pulmonary embolism.

10% of cases will have a 'normal' heart.

The atrial rate is between 350 and 600 beats/min. The AV node will not conduct at this high rate and an irregular ventricular rate will be produced depending on the properties of the AV node but not usually > 200 beats/min.

ECG CHARACTERISTICS (Figure 1)

- Irregular ventricular rate.
- Absent P waves.
- Rapid atrial activity shown as 'F' waves often seen in lead V_1.

Strategies in atrial fibrillation:

- Maintenance of sinus rhythm:

    pro – improved haemodynamics, reduced thrombo-embolic risk

    con – pro-arrhythmic risk, fatality

- Rate control + anticoagulation:

    pro – natural history, avoids pro-arrhythmia

    con – impaired haemodynamics, bleeding, residual embolic risk

Treatment

- Restoration of sinus rhythm is desirable.
- Patients with severe cardiovascular decompensation should be promptly cardioverted electrically.

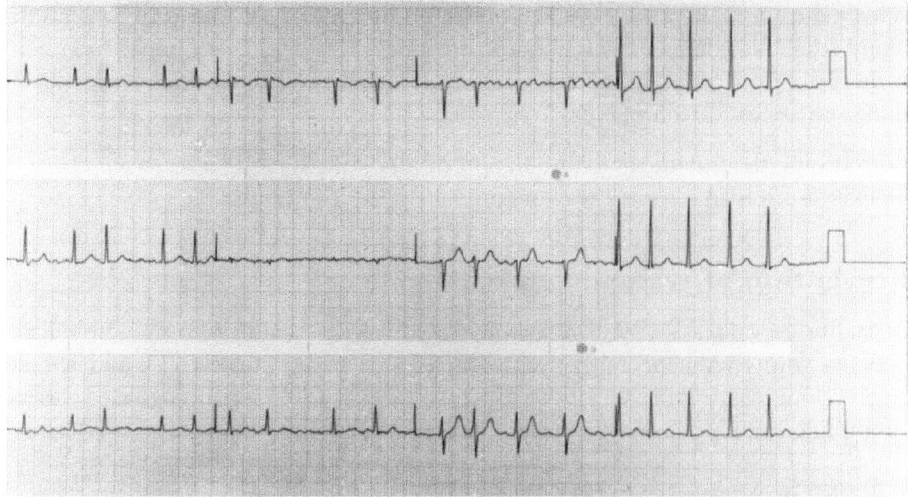

Figure 1

- Patients without ischaemic heart disease can be converted pharmacologically with IV Flecainide (table 3).

- IV amiodarone is also useful in this situation particularly in patients with known ischaemic heart disease.

Patients who have been in atrial fibrillation for > 48 h will need oral anticoagulation for 3–4 weeks before electrical cardioversion.

- Using pressure on the defibrillation paddles and use of the anteroposterior position often increase success.

- For failed external cardioversion, internal cardioversion using relatively low energies will increase the success rate.

If sinus rhythm is not immediately achievable, particularly if the patient has been in atrial fibrillation for some time, then control of the ventricular rate can be

Table 3 – Chemical cardioversion of atrial fibrillation

Highly effective	quinidine
	disopyramide
	flecainide
	propafenone
	aminodarone
Less effective	sotalol
Ineffective	β-blockers
	Calcium antagonists
	digoxin

achieved using a drug to block AV nodal conduction. digoxin has been used for many years but it has a narrow therapeutic index. β-Blockade is a useful treatment if there are no contraindications. Calcium channel blockers such as verapamil or diltiazem are useful alternatives.

For chronic treatment, the combination of digoxin plus a β- or calcium channel blocker is often an effective way of controlling the ventricular rate.

Prevention of systemic embolism

Atrial fibrillation is associated with an increased risk of systemic thrombo-embolism. Patients with rheumatic mitral valve disease are at the greatest risk and should receive long-term anticoagulation. Patients should also be anticoagulated before attempting cardioversion if the patient has been in atrial fibrillation for > 24 h.

Maintenance in sinus rhythm post-cardioversion[3]

The drugs used to maintain sinus rhythm post-cardioversion are:

- Quinidine.
- Flecainide.
- Propafenone.
- Sotalol.
- Amiodarone.
- Defetalide.

Quinidine is effective but associated with excess mortality due to pro-arrhythmic effects. Amiodarone is particularly effective but does have a slow onset of activity and has a relative high incidence of side-effects.

Sinus rhythm can also be achieved in selected patients by a focal ablation of the pulmonary veins or a catheter-based ablation procedure that produce linear burns in the atrium, the so-called catheter maze procedure. These ablation techniques are, however, in their infancy.

ATRIAL FLUTTER

Atrial flutter is associated with the same conditions as atrial fibrillation and is less common. The atria discharge at a rate between 250 and 350 beats/min, the rapid atrial activity reflected by 'F' waves which are regular. These are often associated with no iso-electric line between the F waves having a 'saw tooth' appearance, particularly well seen in lead V_1. There is usually a degree of AV block – most commonly 2:1 AV block – so that the ventricular rate will be 150 beats/min (figure 2). This can often be confused with sinus tachycardia. Accuracy of diagnosis can be improved by blocking AV nodal function either by carotid sinus massage or adenosine, which will reveal atrial flutter waves (figure 3). Typical atrial flutter is also known as common or type 1 atrial flutter as a re-entrant mechanism with the wave front travelling in a counter-clockwise direction in the right atrium. Rapid atrial pacing invariably interrupts the rhythm. Atypical atrial flutter (uncommon or type 2 has a re-entrant wave length travelling in a clockwise direction and cannot be interrupted by atrial pacing).

Treatment

The treatment of sinus rhythm should be the goal as it is difficult to control the ventricular rate with AV nodal blocking drugs.

- Atrial flutter can invariably be terminated by electrical cardioversion at lower energies than with atrial fibrillation. Energies of 25–50 joules are often successful.

- Alternatively, right atrial overdrive pacing is often effective. A temporary pacing lead is inserted into the right atrium and the necessary pacing rate will be between 10 and 30% in excess of the atrial rate. It should be

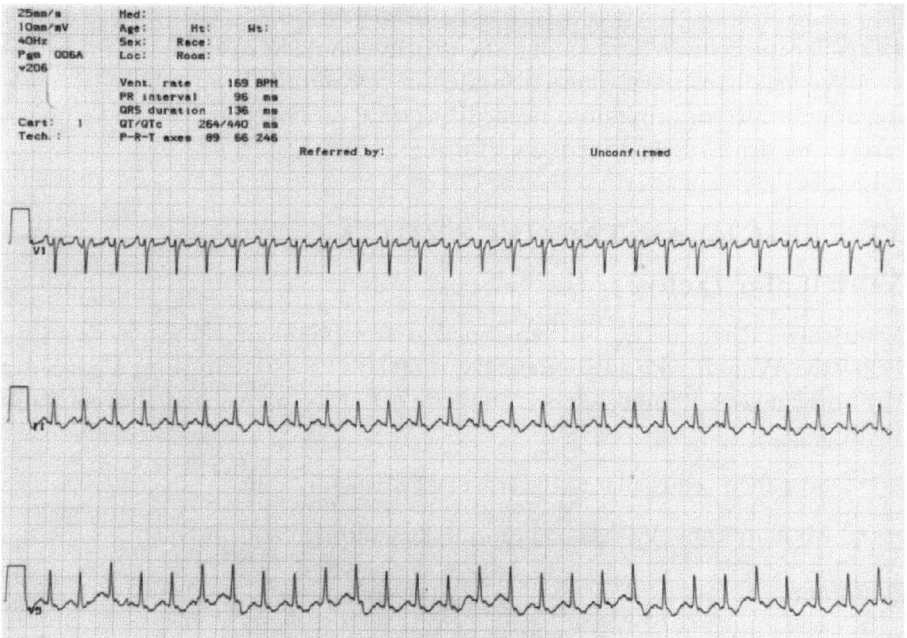

Figure 2

applied for up to 30 s, and on cessation of pacing, sinus rhythm will often return. It is very important to ensure that the pacing lead is in the atrium to guard against rapid ventricular pacing.

- Chemical cardioversion can also be achieved with flecainide and amiodarone.

- Catheter ablation for atrial flutter is now a widely accepted technique with a high incidence of success and can be performed for recurrent flutter not treated by drug therapy.[4]

UNIFOCAL ATRIAL TACHYCARDIA

- Arises from atrial muscle that does not include sinus node.

- Characterized by single P wave morphology (atrial rate < 250 beats/min).

- Tends to be incessant rather than paroxysmal.

- Important cause of tachycardia-related cardiomyopathy.

- Occasionally secondary to digoxin toxicity usually with 2:1 or 3:1 AV block.

Treatment

In a patient receiving treatment digoxin, toxicity should be suspected. If the patient is not taking digoxin, the ventricular rate can be controlled with AV nodal blocking drugs or, if sinus rhythm is needed, electrical cardioversion should be undertaken. Overdrive atrial pacing is a useful alternative.

VENTRICULAR TACHYCARDIAS

Ventricular tachycardia

Ventricular tachycardia is usually defined as 4 or more consecutive beats arising below the AV node with a RR interval of < 500 ms (> 120 beats/min). Ventricular rhythms between 100 and 120 beats/min are defined as accelerated idioventricular rhythm.

- Sustained ventricular tachycardia (VT) lasts for > 30 s.

- Monomorphic VT has one morphology during each episode.

Aetiology

- Myocardial ischaemia (acute or chronic).

- Dilated cardiomyopathy.

- Hypertrophic cardiomyopathy.

- Myocarditis.

- Right ventricular dysplasia.

- Drug toxicity.

- Electrolyte abnormality.

ECG criteria (figure 4)

- ECG criteria have been established for the diagnosis of VT in the presence of a wide QRS tachycardia (QRS > 120 ms). The criteria are used in particular to distinguish this arrhythmia from supraventricular tachycardia with aberrant conduction.

- In general, the QRS duration is longer in VT than in supraventricular tachycardia with aberrant conduction (QRS duration > 140 ms of tachycardias with a right bundle branch block morphology; > 160 ms of tachycardias with a left bundle branch block morphology).

- The most useful reliable criterion is the presence of AV dissociation. This independent atrial activity is often seen in lead II. Intermittent capture of the ventricles by conduction from independent atrial activity (capture beat), narrow QRS or fusion beats (shape intermediate between sinus and tachycardia morphologies) are good markers for VT. Positive concordance of QRS complexes in the chest leads (i.e. prominent deflection of each QRS complex is positive).

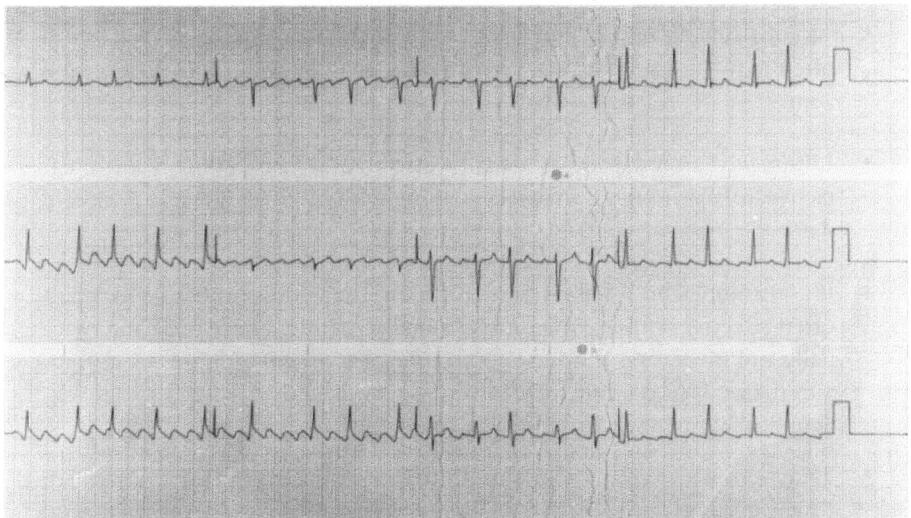

Figure 3

- The absence of an RS complex in all precordial leads, or if an RS complex is present in one of more precordial leads, an RS interval which is broad (> 100 ms) is highly specific of VT.

A pre-existing 12-lead ECG would provide useful information. If a bundle branch block is present in sinus rhythm with a different morphology or axis to that during the tachycardia then the tachycardia is very likely to be ventricular in origin. If d waves are present on the surface ECG, the diagnosis is most probably that of WPW with antidromic AVRT or pre-excited atrial fibrillation. In atrial fibrillation the rhythm will also be irregular.

If the patient is stable and there is still diagnostic difficulty, then IV adenosine can be a useful diagnostic tool. Adenosine will terminate the supraventricular tachycardia. The vast majority of ventricular tachycardias will not be affected by adenosine. An exception to this rule is of fascicular tachycardia.

It is important not to give verapamil for a broad complex tachycardia due to the incidence of life-threatening hypotension associated with its administration in VT.

Treatment

- VT with haemodynamic compromise necessitates prompt electrical cardioversion.

- IV lignocaine 100 mg is a useful first-line drug but will only be effective in about 30% of cases.

- Amiodarone IV is extremely effective and has a long onset of action often requiring at least 900–1200 mg/day as an IV infusion into a central vein.

- Ultimately amiodarone is usually effective at controlling ventricular tachycardia although it may take loading with up to 20 g over a period of days.

- If controlling the VT is proving difficult, the addition of a β-blocker is often effective, either using sotalol alone at an initial dose of 80 mg twice daily and increasing it up to a total daily dose of 480 mg if necessary. An alternative is a combination of amiodarone and a β-blocker such as atenolol 50 mg/day.

- Transvenous pacing is also a useful treatment to terminate a VT when drugs are ineffective or the VT is recurrent. A burst of overdrive right ventricular pacing is often successful in terminating a tachycardia.

It is also important to treat the underlying cause if at all possible, i.e. correct electrolyte abnormalities and hypoxia. Patients with recurrent VT, which is not responding to therapy, should be discussed with a tertiary cardiological centre. If the underlying substrate for the ventricular tachycardia is ischaemia, then revascularization either by coronary artery surgery or coronary intervention should be considered. Some patients will also require electrophysiological study with a view to either ablative therapy or the insertion of an implantable defibrillator.

Polymorphic ventricular tachycardia

- Characterized by repeated progressive change in the QRS complex so that the complexes appear to 'twist' around the base line.

- Often seen associated with a prolongation of the QT interval when it is called torsade de pointes.[5]

Causes of torsade de pointes include:

- Congenital long QT syndrome (LQTS).

- Hypokalaemia.

- Ischaemia.

- Anti-arrhythmic drugs.

- Tricyclic antidepressants.

- Bradycardia (sick sinus syndrome or AV block).

Treatment

Management should be guided to the underlying cause. Congenital prolongation of a QT interval is often associated with VT. This tachycardia is usually induced by sympathetic over-activity either by inversion or extremes of emotion. It can cause syncope or even sudden death. Treatment is with β-blockade (the long-acting β-blocker nadolol is particularly useful). Many patients need implantable cardiac defibrillators.

- Cases secondary to ischaemia should have the substrate changed by revascularization.

- Pacing is the treatment of choice for bradycardia.

- Anti-arrhythmic drugs that produce this arrhythmia either alone or in combination should be withdrawn.

- IV magnesium will suppress the acquired form of torsade de pointes.

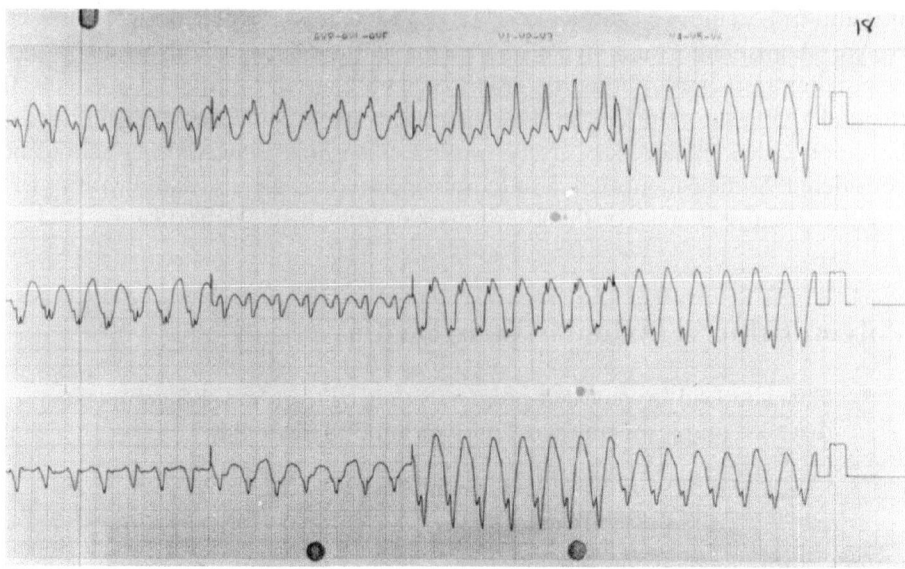

Figure 4

Ventricular fibrillation

Ventricular fibrillation is a rapid totally incoordinate contraction of ventricular myocardial fibres reflected in the ECG by chaotic electrical activity. It is associated with circulatory arrest. The vast majority of cases are secondary to myocardial ischaemia particularly myocardial infarction and is the commonest form of death in acute MI. Treatment is with prompt defibrillation.

- When associated with acute MI, VF is most common during the first hour of the onset of chest pain.

- When ventricular fibrillation is not associated with myocardial infarction or ischaemia, i.e. 'primary VF', full investigation and referral to a tertiary cardiological centre is mandatory as the patient will invariably need an implantable defibrillator.

Atrioventricular block

- Atrioventricular (AV) is classified as first, second or third degree. This depends on whether the conduction of atrial impulses to the ventricle is delayed, intermittently blocked or blocked completely.

- Second-degree AV block is subdivided into Mobitz I (Wenckebach) and II types. Mobitz I is associated with progressive lengthening of the PR interval before a non-conduction of atrial impulse. In Mobitz II AV block, the PR interval is constant.

There are many causes of AV block including:

- Idiopathic fibrosis.

- Ischaemia.

- Aortic valve disease.

- Cardiac surgery.

- Infiltration.

- Inflammation.

- Rheumatic fever.

Treatment is not needed for first-degree heart block. Patients will invariably require pacing for second- and third-degree AV block. The indications are discussed in Chapter 9.

Sick sinus syndrome (sino-atrial disease)

The syndrome is due to abnormal sinus node activity resulting in sinus bradycardia, sino-atrial block or sinus arrest. It is often associated with tachycardias of supraventricular origin, usually atrial fibrillation and is then often called 'bradycardia tachycardia syndrome'. The underlying cause is usually idiopathic fibrosis of the sinus node.

Treatment is usually with permanent pacing. Further details and indications are given in Chapter 9.

Further reading

Akhtar M, Shenasa M, Jazayeri *et al.* Wide QRS complex tachycardia: reappraisal of a common clinical problem. *Ann Intern Med* 1988; **109**: 905–12.

Morganroth J, Bigger JT. Pharmacologic management of ventricular arrhythmias after the Cardiac Arrhythmia Suppression Trial. *Am J Cardiol* 1990; **65**: 1497–503.

Singh BN. Controlling cardiac arrhythmias: an overview with a historical perspective. *Am J Cardiol* 1997: **80**; 4G–15G.

References

1. Packer DL, Bardy GH, Worley SJ *et al.* Tachycardia-induced cardiomyopathy: a reversible form of left ventricular dysfunction. *Am J Cardiol* 1986; **57**: 563–70.

2. Griffiths MJ, Linker NJ, Ward DE, Camm AJ. Adenosine in the diagnosis of broad complex tachycardia. *Lancet* 1988; **i**: 672–5.

3. Crijins HJ, van Gelder IC. Serial antiarrhythmic drug treatment to maintain sinus rhythm after electrical cardioversion for chronic atrial fibrillation or atrial flutter. *Am J Cardiol* 1991; **68**; 335–41.

4. Kuck KH, Schl ter M, Geiger M *et al.* Radiofrequency current catheter ablation of accessory atrioventricular pathways. *Lancet* 1991; **337**: 1557–61.

5. Ben-David J, Zipes DP. Torsade de pointes and proarrhythmia. *Lancet* 1993; **341**; 1578–82.

16

MISCELLANEOUS EMERGENCIES

HYPERTENSIVE EMERGENCIES

Hypertension is one of the major risk factors for the development of coronary cerebral and renovascular diseases and its presence in Western societies is reaching almost endemic proportions. Fortunately the large numbers of patients involved are not translated into a high incidence of true hypertensive emergencies.

WHAT CONSTITUTES A HYPERTENSIVE EMERGENCY?

- Malignant or accelerated hypertension is the term given to a very high diastolic blood pressure (traditionally > 130 mmHg).

- Sustained blood pressures of this degree are often associated with acute vascular damage. This is usually manifest by retinal changes; haemorrhages and exudates (grade III retinopathy), and/or papilloedema (grade IV retinopathy), heart failure or encephalopathy (headache, irritability, alteration in consciousness, fits or fluctuating neurological signs).

- Malignant hypertension may also be associated with renal dysfunction, manifest by protein and red cells in the urine or by renal failure. Elevated renin levels result in secondary aldosteronism and may produce hypokalaemia (sometimes mistaken as being indicative of primary aldosteronism causing the hypertensive crisis). Micro-angiopathic haemolytic anaemia and disseminated intravascular coagulation can occur.

- Patients may have very few signs or symptoms despite having severely elevated blood pressure; however, they should also be treated actively as the prognosis of untreated hypertension of this degree is very poor (75% mortality rate at 1 year).

- Occasionally patients with blood pressures lower than this may need emergency reduction of blood pressure (table 1).

- Rarely blood pressures can be elevated to the 'malignant' level in acute anxiety states and this must not be mistaken for a hypertensive emergency. But bear in mind that the cerebral dysfunction of malignant hypertension may mimic some features of an acute anxiety state.

Treatment

- Before deciding on therapy a distinction has to be made between those patients who need emergency reduction of blood pressure and those who need less rapid but still urgent treatment. It is a common misconception that all patients with blood pressures in the malignant range need parenteral therapy.

- Emergency therapy (usually parenteral) is indicated in all patients with hypertensive encephalopathy, in patients who are at immediate danger from continuing high blood pressure (table 1) and in those in whom oral therapy is not working or is unlikely to work (e.g. pheochromocytoma).

- Urgent therapy (usually oral) generally produces a satisfactory response in patients who are alert and in little obvious distress.

- Rapid reductions in blood pressure can be dangerous and subsequent tissue ischaemia can lead to stroke, blindness and myocardial infarction. In those patients who present with a stroke and coincidentally raised blood pressure, rapid reductions in blood pressure can produce further

Table 1 Circumstance requiring urgent (often parenteral) lowering of blood pressure.

Cardiovascular
> Acute aortic dissection
> Acute left ventricular failure
> After coronary bypass surgery

Cerebrovascular
> Hypertensive encephalopathy
> Intracerebral haemorrhage
> Subarachnoid haemorrhage

Miscellaneous
> Pheochromocytoma crisis
> Head injury

cerebral ischaemia and can be fatal! Deciding whether the neurological features on admission are indicative of hypertensive encephalopathy or a cerebrovascular accident can be very difficult. The following factors must be borne in mind:

- hypertensive encephalopathy is exceedingly rare, whereas cerebrovascular accidents are common

- hypertensive encephalopathy often produces fluctuating neurological features

- Other signs of malignant hypertension are usually present.

Parenteral treatment

If parenteral therapy is required there are currently two recommended drugs: sodium nitroprusside and labetolol. They should both only be administered in an intensive care or high-dependency unit where facilities for intensive monitoring exist.

If the patient presents with encephalopathy or heart failure the drug of choice is nitroprusside. This acts as an arteriolar and venous dilator thereby reducing venous return and cardiac output, its dilatory properties may actually increase cerebral blood flow and potentially exacerbate the encephalopathic picture. However, its speed of action and potency mean that blood pressure reduction negates these adverse effects.

- Sodium nitroprusside is given by continuous infusion starting at 0.5 μg/kg/min, increasing to 8 μg/kg/min according to response (nitroprusside is photodegraded by sunlight and must be covered by reflective foil, new solutions must be prepared every 4 h). Its speed of action is instantaneous so very careful monitoring of blood pressure is required. Ideally this should be by intra-arterial monitoring, but if this is not available then the blood pressure should be taken every 60 s until a steady-state is reached. **(Note: some automated blood pressure cuffs may give inaccurate readings at very high blood pressures and manual readings should supplement these recordings.)** The aim should be to lower the diastolic blood pressure to no lower than 100–110 mmHg. Oral therapy must be started as soon as possible and this may require more than one drug. After the institution of oral therapy the nitroprusside should be gradually weaned, to do this too rapidly or before oral medication has taken effect can result in rebound hypertension.

- Labetalol is a β-blocker with some α-antagonist activity at higher doses; its speed of action is 5–10 min and therefore it may take slightly longer to reach a steady-state and fine control is not as easy as with nitroprusside. Its use is contraindicated in patients with heart failure and asthma. It should be infused at 1–3 mg/min, with the same aims as above. Once again, oral drug therapy should be established before titrating down the dose.

There seems to be a trend particularly in some A&E departments to treat hypertension with IV isosorbide dinitrate. While this may be beneficial in patients with heart failure, its vasodilatory action may worsen an encephalopathic crisis and its antihypertensive properties may not be sufficient to compensate.

Oral therapy

While conservative therapy has no place to play in the management of severe hypertension, some drop in blood pressure may be seen with bed rest. Oral therapy is preferable to parenteral therapy as the reductions in blood pressure are often more gradual, thus avoiding the acute ischaemic complications. When not contraindicated, a β-blocker such as atenolol 50–100 mg should be used. Nifedipine 10–20 mg, methyl-dopa 250 mg or hydralazine 25 mg are suitable alternatives. It is probably best to avoid ACE inhibitors in the acute phase because of the possibility of renal involvement in the hypertensive process, but their use can be considered later in the treatment schedule. If the first dose fails to reduce the blood pressure sufficiently then a second dose can be given 4 h later. The aim should be to reduce the diastolic pressure to 110 mmHg over the first 12 h. Further control over the next few days often requires more than one drug.

Properly managed hypertensive emergencies can result in a dramatic improvement in survival in the acute situation with survival rates of 90% at 1 year and 80% at 5 years. Death in patients with severe hypertension usually results from stroke or renal failure if it occurs in the first few years, or from ischaemic heart disease if they survive this period.

Aortic dissection

Dissection of the thoracic aorta is one of the most feared presentations of any acute medical emergencies. This stems from the fact that the condition is often not easy to diagnose and the consequences for misdiagnosis are dire.

Unfortunately the condition is relatively common and there are > 2000 new cases/year in the USA.[1] There is a male:female ratio of 2:1 and its peak incidence is in 60–70-year-olds, although it can occur at any age. It is thought to arise from medial degeneration of the aortic wall. This usually occurs as a result of chronic shear stresses often exacerbated by hypertension, but can be an intrinsic defect of collagen tissue, such as occurs in Marfans and Ehlers–Danlos syndromes.

A surgical perspective on this condition is provided in Chapter 17.

Presentation

- The presentation in an individual patient depends on the path and extent of the dissection. Pain is the usual presenting symptom, characteristically being extremely severe and described (somewhat helpfully) as 'tearing' or 'ripping'. Most texts state that the pain is felt in the intrascapular area. However, if the dissection is confined to the ascending aorta the pain may be felt only retrosternally or in the neck or jaw.[2] The pain may also migrate.

- Other presenting symptoms include heart failure, neurological signs mimicking cerebrovascular accidents, ischaemic limbs and syncope (it has been reported if the latter is present cardiac tamponade may have occurred).[2]

- The blood pressure is frequently elevated. If low, tamponade may have occurred, or dissection of a brachiocephalic artery may be producing 'pseudo-hypotension'.

- The sign of differential blood pressures in the upper limbs will only occur if the dissection only involves and impedes the flow of one of the supplying arteries, the sign may also be transient. While more common in proximal than distal dissections, the sign should not be relied on solely as the much commoner atherosclerotic narrowing of these vessels often produces it.

- Aortic regurgitation is a very important sign to elicit, and may be present in up to 50% of proximal dissections.[3] When present it usually indicates involvement of the valvular apparatus in the dissecting process. However, aortic regurgitation can predate the dissection and occur as a result of aortic root dilation secondary to hypertension.

- If signs of heart failure are present it is usually due to the onset of severe aortic regurgitation.

- Pleural effusions may result from rupture of the aorta or as a result of an acute inflammatory response.

- Many more signs can be present and are predictable either on the direct involvement of a vascular supply or by direct compression.

Investigation

If aortic dissection is suspected urgent investigation is required. Chest X-ray may reveal a dilated aorta, cardiac enlargement (if a pericardial effusion is present) and the presence of a pleural effusion. The classical appearances of an acute myocardial infarction may occur on an ECG due to dissection of one of the coronary artery ostia. Caution must therefore be exercised in treating this along conventional lines, as administration of thrombolytic therapy will prove rapidly fatal. However, there are four main diagnostic imaging modalities:

- Echocardiography – transthoracic echocardiography can reveal the presence of aortic regurgitation, dilated aortic root, presence of pericardial fluid and occasionally a dissection flap in the ascending aorta. However, transoesophageal echocardiography gives much better visualization of the aortic root and valve, as well as excellent views of the descending aorta. This is now widely regarded as the investigation of choice as its sensitivity and specificity have been quoted at 99 and 98% respectively.[4] The only disadvantage is that the lower limit of extensive dissections may not be defined. Some centres, including ours, recommend that in acutely ill cases or in cases where there is a high probability of type A dissection this should be carried out in the anaesthetic room of the cardiothoracic theatre, where rapid surgical intervention can be carried out if necessary. This latter safeguard is obviously only possible in a cardiothoracic centre and thus where these facilities do not exist it may be necessary to perform the investigation before transferring the patient for surgery. The overriding priority should be to make the diagnosis as quickly and safely as possible.

- Computed tomography – CT visualization of a dissection requires the injection of contrast, but it has the advantage of being able to image the whole aorta. It will provide no information on aortic regurgitation.

- Magnetic resonance imaging (MRI) – gives excellent visualization of the whole aorta without the need for contrast. Its main disadvantage is that access to an acutely ill patient is impaired and special monitoring and therapeutic equipment is required.

- Cardiac catheterization – used to be the investigation of choice as it gives good visualization of the whole aorta, although often two imaging planes are required to see asymmetrical dissections. It also has the advantage of imaging the coronary arteries that are often involved in the atherosclerotic process. However, it is now generally recommended that this invasive procedure is not carried out as it often delays surgery and increases mortality rates.

Treatment

This is aimed at halting the progression of the dissection and treating the complications that have already arisen. Without therapy the mortality rate is 25% at 24 h, 50% at 1 week, 75% at 1 month and 90% at 1 year.[4] If aortic regurgitation or tamponade has occurred, the mortality rate approaches 100% within a few hours.

Surgery

- Required for all type A dissections (provided co-morbid conditions allow).

- Required for complications – vital organ involvement, rupture or imminent rupture and aortic dissection.

- Required for Marfans' syndrome.

- Often very complicated involving repair of the dissection flap and aortic root replacement with or without aortic valve replacement.

- Complication rates are high including cerebral ischaemia and paraplegia caused by ischaemia of the spinal or intercostal arteries.

- Survival rates of 80–90% are reported.[5]

Medical

- Advised for type B dissections.

- Advised for all chronic dissections (> 2 weeks after onset of dissection) because of universally poor prognosis.

- Advised for patients who have co-morbid conditions prohibiting surgery.

- All patients with suspected dissection should be treated medically until the diagnosis is made.

- Medical therapy consists of lowering the blood pressure to 100–110 mmHg systolic. This is often best performed using labetolol often in combination with sodium nitroprusside in the same way as described above for the management of malignant hypertension. If β-blockers are contraindicated, calcium antagonists such as verapamil may be useful. Oral therapy should be instituted as soon as possible in those continuing with medical therapy.

ENDOCARDITIS

Some would question the inclusion of endocarditis in a handbook of cardiac emergencies; however, delay in treatment can often result in marked progression of the disease process and consequently produce more severe cardiac compromise. It is most commonly caused by bacterial infection but fungal infections can occur. Occasionally no organism can be identified – 'culture-negative endocarditis' will be discussed below.

Presentation

- In its florid forms infective endocarditis produces a typical picture of fluctuating fever, malaise, weight loss, night sweats in association with a heart murmur.

- Often, however, the picture is less florid and presentation is very insidious, often mimicking many other illnesses.

- One of the complications of endocarditis may be the presenting feature (see below).

Diagnosis

- Based on the Duke clinical criteria (table 2).

Table 2 Duke clinical criteria for the diagnosis of infective endocarditits (IE)

Major criteria

1. Positive blood cultures :

A. Typical organism consistent with IE from 2 separate blood cultures:
    (i) viridans streptococci, strep bovis, or HACEK (Actinobacillus actinomycetemcomitans, Cardiobacterium hominus, Eikenella corrodens, and kingella sp.) group
    (ii) community acquired staph aureus or enterococci in the absence of a primary focus.

B. Organisms consistent with IE from persistently positive blood cultures :
    (i) >2 positive blood cultures >12 hours apart
    (ii) all of 3 or the majority of >4 blood cultures >1 hour apart.

2. Evidence of endocardial involvement

A. Positive echocardiogram:
(i) oscillating intracardiac mass on valve or supporting structures, in the path of regurgitant jets, or on implanted material in the absence of an alternative anatomic explanation
(ii) abscess
(iii) new partial dehiscence of prosthetic valve
B. New valvular regurgitation

Minor criteria (Nos. 7 and 8 not in the original classification)
1. Predisposition
2. Fever >38C
3. Vascular phenomena
4. Immunological phenomena
5. Microbiological evidence not meeting major criteria, or serology
6. Echocardiographic evidence consistent with IE not meeting major criteria
(7. Elevated ESR or c-reactive protein)
(8. Newly diagnosed clubbing, splenomegaly, microscopic haematuria)

- Using this criteria endocarditis is classified as definite, possible or rejected (table 3).

- From tables 2 and 3 it is obvious that microbiology has a major part to play in the diagnosis. Currently it is recommended that at least three pairs of blood cultures (aerobic and anaerobic) are taken from three different sites over the course of about 1 h **before** commencing antibiotic therapy.

- A high index of suspicion is required to prevent cases being overlooked. Patients with prosthetic valves, with pre-existing cardiac defects that predispose to the development of endocarditis and IV drug users should have all pyrexias considered as being potentially caused by endocarditis and have blood cultures taken.

- Echocardiography is also the mainstay of diagnosis. In suspected cases a transthoracic scan should be carried out as soon as possible. This only has a sensitivity of 50–60% and in suspected cases with a negative scan it is necessary to perform a transoesophageal echocardiogram. The sensitivity and specificity of this investigation has been reported as 98 and 99% respectively.[6]

Table 3 Diagnosis of infective endocarditis

Definite

Pathological criteria:

(i) Micro-organisms: demonstrated by culture of histology in a vegetation or abscess
(ii) Pathological lesions: vegetation or intracardiac abscess present confirmed by histology showing active endocarditis

Clinical criteria:

(i) 2 Major criteria
(ii) 1 Major and 3 minor criteria
(iii) 5 Minor criteria

Possible

Not definite or rejected

Rejected

(i) Firm alternative diagnosis
(ii) Resolution of manifestations with antibiotics for <4 days
(iii) No pathological evidence at surgery or post mortem after <4 days antibiotics

- In the authors' view transoesophageal echocardiography should also be performed in all cases where endocarditis has been confirmed on transthoracic scanning because of the much higher detection rate of cardiac complications.

- Diagnosis is occasionally very difficult and in this scenario it is necessary to continue repeating blood cultures and often repeating the transthoracic (and occasionally transoesophageal) echo after a few weeks.

Treatment

- Treatment of infective endocarditis must be commenced with high-dose IV antibiotics as soon as possible. However, it is important to obtain blood for culture before the first dose of antibiotics.

- Blind therapy is based on the likely causative organism. In the vast majority of cases this will be streptococcal, enterococcal or staphylococcal, and the most common starting regimen is: benzylpenicillin up to 12 g by 4-hourly divided doses in 24 h; flucloxacillin up to 6 g by 4–6-hourly divided doses in 24 h; gentamicin up to 240 mg in 8–12-hourly divided doses in 24 h.

- Discussion with a microbiologist at the earliest possible opportunity is essential in **every** suspected case as the antibiotic regimen should be individualized for each patient.

- Culture reports should guide antibiotic therapy as should the patients clinical response.

- Antibiotic therapy should be continued for 6 weeks where possible. However, some authorities suggest that in uncomplicated cases the final 2 weeks of this may be with oral antibiotics.

- Some patients will need surgical intervention to deal with or prevent complications of endocarditis. In some this may be required before the completion of the antibiotic course. It is best to have as long a course of antibiotics as possible before intervening as this reduces the risk of subsequent infection on any implanted prosthetic material.

Complications

Congestive cardiac failure

- Occurs with the aortic valve more frequently than the mitral valve, which occurs more frequently than tricuspid valve infections.

- Can occur acutely due to chordal rupture, valve perforation or obstruction.

- More often insidious due to gradual worsening of leaks and left ventricular dilation.

- When it has occurred the surgical risks increase and long-term prognosis decreases.

Embolization

- Occurs in 22–50% of cases.

- Can cause ischaemia of supplied territory. Most often this is cerebral and the middle cerebral artery territory is particularly often affected.

- Occurs most often with infections by *Staphylococcus aureus* and *Candida*.

- Mitral valve vegetations embolize more frequently than aortic valve vegetations.

Periannular extension

- An ominous feature and predicts a higher mortality rate, the development of CCF.

- More common in aortic valve endocarditis and IV drug users.

- Its presence may be predicted by the development of new heart block on an ECG, which is caused by the involvement of the electrical conducting system.

Abscess

- Most commonly splenic but any organ may be affected.

Mycotic aneurysms

- Can occur in any vascular structure.

- Often require surgical repair as have a tendency to rupture.

Culture-negative endocarditis

- Fortunately true culture-negative endocarditis is uncommon (< 5% of cases).

- The incidence of false-negative cultures can occur due to inadequate or inappropriate microbiological techniques, as occasionally prolonged culture and enrichment techniques are required. This fault often arises when the microbiology department has not been informed about the clinical suspicions.

- Organisms causing endocarditis can be difficult to culture or require special techniques to isolate (HACEK, *Brucella*, *Legionella*, *Coxiella*, *Chlamydia* and fungi).

- Patients who have recently received antibiotics reduce isolation rates by 30–40%.

- Endocarditis rarely may not have an infective origin as in marantic endocarditis, which occurs in association with a systemic malignancy, or in Libman–Sacks endocarditis with systemic lupus erythematosus.

Further reading

Bayer AS, Bolger AF, Taubert KA *et al*. Diagnosis and management of infective endocarditis and its complications. *Circulation* 1998; **98**: 2936–48.

Eagle KA, De Sanctis RW. Diseases of the aorta. In Braunwald E (ed.), *Heart Disease*. Philadelphia: WB Saunders, 1992: 1528–57.

References

1. Wheat MW. Acute dissecting aneurysms of the aorta: diagnosis and treatment. *Am Heart J* 1980; **99**: 373.

2. Slater EE, DeSanctis RW. The clinical recognition of dissecting aortic aneurysm. *Am Med J* 1976; **60**: 625.

3. Erbel R, Engberding R, Daniel W *et al*. Echocardiography in diagnosis of aortic dissection. *Lancet* 1989; **i**: 457.

4. Anagnostopoulos CE, Prabhakar MJS, Kittle CF. Aortic dissections and dissecting aneurysms. *Am J Cardiol* 1972; **30**: 263.

5. Glower DD, Fann JI, Speier RH *et al*. Comparison of medical and surgical therapy for uncomplicated descending aortic dissection. *Circulation* 1989; **80 (suppl. II)**: 24.

6. Bayer AS, Bolger AF, Taubert KA *et al*. Diagnosis and management of infective endocarditis and its complications. *Circulation* 1998; **98**: 2936–48.

17

ROLE OF SURGICAL
INTERVENTION

For the purposes of this chapter, emergencies are defined as conditions that require surgical intervention without any delay, regardless of the time of day, as opposed to urgent conditions which require surgery within the same hospital admission.[1] Table 1 lists various cardiac surgical emergencies and defines the scope of this chapter.

EMERGENCIES ASSOCIATED WITH ISCHAEMIC HEART DISEASE

Unstable angina

Unstable angina is a medical emergency and its clinical presentation and management have been discussed in Chapter 14. Most patients with unstable angina should be managed medically; > 90% will stabilize.[2] Those with persistent symptoms despite full medical therapy require urgent coronary angiography with a view

Table 1 – Cardiac surgical emergencies.

Emergencies associated with ischaemic heart disease
•   Unstable angina
•   Mechanical complications of myocardial infarction
Emergencies associated with valvular heart disease
•   Acute mitral regurgitation
•   Bacterial endocarditis
•   Mechanical complications of prosthetic heart valves
Other cardiac surgical emergencies
•   Aortic dissection
•   Cardiac trauma
•   Cardiac tamponade
•   Massive pulmonary embolism
•   Mechanical cardiac support

to percutaneous intervention or coronary artery bypass surgery. Indications for emergency coronary artery bypass in patients with unstable angina are rare,[3] but include the following in patients who are unsuitable for angioplasty or in whom angioplasty has failed:

- Prolonged ongoing (> 20 min) rest pain despite maximal medical therapy including IV nitrates.

- Continuing evidence of ischaemia on ECG.

- Ischaemic left ventricular failure.

- Angina with hypotension.

- Angina with new or worsening mitral regurgitant murmur.

- Refractory unstable post-infarction angina.

Patients with the above features are at high risk of death or non-fatal infarction in the short-term.[4]

MECHANICAL COMPLICATIONS OF ACUTE MYOCARDIAL INFARCTION (SEE ALSO CHAPTER 12)

- Acute mitral regurgitation.

- Post-infarction ventricular septal defect.

- Pseudo-aneurysm.

Acute mitral regurgitation

Acute mitral regurgitation is an uncommon but serious complication of acute myocardial infarction that may occur as a result of chordal or papillary muscle rupture, with leaflet prolapse. The left atrium remains small and the regurgitant wave is transmitted directly to the pulmonary veins, with pulmonary hypertension, sudden onset of dyspnoea and acute pulmonary oedema, most commonly 2–7 days after the acute infarction. In total rupture of a papillary muscle, cardiogenic shock may result. A new, loud pansystolic murmur at the apex or left sternal edge should alert the clinician to the diagnosis, although this is absent in total rupture. There may be an associated thrill. Even when present, the murmur is easily missed due to tachycardia, gallop rhythm and diffuse crepitations or rhonchi from pulmonary oedema. Chest X-ray may also be misleading, with bilateral whiteouts mimicking pneumonia. Echocardiography confirms the diagnosis, which should be followed by urgent left ventricular and coronary angiography, the latter to delineate coronary anatomy.

Management

Only about 25% of patients survive > 24 h after total rupture of a papillary muscle. Fulminant pulmonary oedema with haemodynamic collapse requires admission to the intensive care unit for invasive monitoring and ventilatory and inotropic support. An intra-aortic balloon pump should be inserted to provide mechanical cardiac assist. Emergency mitral valve repair or replacement with concomitant coronary artery bypass grafting may be life saving. Although the operative mortality rate is high, late results are good in survivors, with most patients in NYHA class I or II 3–5 years after surgery. Partial rupture with less severe mitral regurgitation may be managed initially by medical therapy, although all patients should undergo urgent surgery during the same hospital admission.

Post-infarction ventricular septal defect

This is a catastrophic complication of acute myocardial infarction with a mortality rate of 50% in the first week and 80% at 4 weeks without surgical treatment. Traditionally the onset is 7–10 days post-infarction, but following thrombolysis septal rupture may occur as early as 3 days post-infarction.[5] Low output failure rather than acute pulmonary oedema dominate the clinical picture, and right-sided signs are prominent in the early stages, with very high venous pressures. Physical signs may be very similar to chordal or papillary muscle rupture, but echocardiography is diagnostic.

Management

Large post-infarction VSD frequently progress to cardiogenic shock, with hypotension, renal failure and cerebral obtundation. Admission to the coronary care unit for invasive monitoring and inotropic support is required. Insertion of an intra-aortic balloon pump is beneficial. Emergency repair of the VSD with concomitant coronary artery bypass may be life-saving, although surgical mortality in the presence of cardiogenic shock is > 30%. Patients with anterior infarction and good right ventricular function do better.[6] Medium term results are disappointing: overall, only 40% of patients survive 5 years. Nevertheless, survivors are usually symptomatically well and in NYHA class I or II. Of those who die, most die of cardiac-related causes.

Not all patients with post-infarction VSD require emergency surgery. Those with moderate shunts should be stabilized with inotropic and vasodilator therapy, and intra-aortic balloon support. This may allow surgery remote from the acute infarction, with a correspondingly lower operative risk. Patients with small acquired VSD may tolerate their condition well with little haemodynamic upset. If possible, they should wait 6 weeks to allow cicatrization of the edges of the VSD before surgery.

Pseudoaneurysm

Free ventricular rupture following myocardial infarction is usually fatal and presents with acute cardiac tamponade and sudden death. Occasionally subacute cardiac rupture occurs in which adhesions to the pericardium forms a barrier to free rupture, with pseudo-aneurysm formation. Such aneurysms have a narrow mouth, and a strong tendency to rupture.[7] Resection with repair of the ventricular defect is clearly advisable.

EMERGENCIES ASSOCIATED WITH VALVULAR HEART DISEASE

Acute mitral regurgitation

Acute mitral regurgitation may also occur as a result of chordal rupture in myxomatous degeneration, or endocarditis. Despite the presence of severe mitral regurgitation, physical examination often reveals preservation of sinus rhythm. The murmur is more ejection in quality and sometimes mid-to-late systolic, and may be best heard at the left sternal edge (posterior chordal rupture) or at the back (anterior chordal rupture). Echocardiography is diagnostic. Medical treatment including intensive vasodilator (see Chapter 2) therapy may hold the situation temporarily; insertion of an intra-aortic balloon pump is beneficial. However, the prognosis is poor without surgery and emergency mitral valve repair or replacement should be considered.

Bacterial endocarditis

This topic is covered in detail in Chapter 16. Valvular destruction with progressive aortic or mitral incompetence may result in haemodynamic compromise and worsening heart failure. In such circumstances urgent, rather than emergency, surgery is indicated. Urgent surgery should also be considered if:

- the infection is refractory to antibiotic therapy
- there is aortic regurgitation with progressive subannular infection, e.g. aneurysm, abscess or fistulation
- there is worsening prolongation of AV conduction
- there is a recurrent embolic phenomenon

In neglected cases, catastrophic valve failure may necessitate emergency surgery.

MECHANICAL COMPLICATIONS OF PROSTHETIC HEART VALVES

Failure of prosthetic heart valves is an uncommon but potentially catastrophic complication that constitutes a genuine cardiac surgical emergency. The mode of failure depends on the type of prosthesis. The majority of bioprostheses fail as a result of degenerative calcification and leaflet tear with incompetence of the affected valve (74% of explanted bioprostheses), while thrombosis is the dominant cause of mechanical valve dysfunction (18% of failures).[8]

The incidence of primary tissue failure in biological valves is time-related: in the first 7 years after implantation structural failure is uncommon and occurs at 1–2%/patient-year. The failure rate then increases rapidly and is age- and position-dependent: at 10 years in the aortic position, 35% of patients < 60 years old will have undergone re-operation for structural failure, as compared with 10% of patients > 60 years old. In the mitral position, the corresponding figures are 50% for patients < 60 years old and 25% for patients > 60 years old. Primary tissue failure of biological prostheses generally leads to progressive valvular dysfunction, which allows elective re-operation with an acceptable operative risk. Uncommonly, acute leaflet rupture results in precipitous haemodynamic deterioration that necessitates emergency surgery, with a correspondingly high operative mortality rate (30–40%).

Thrombotic valve dysfunction occurs when thrombotic deposits interfere with the valve mechanism, preventing full opening or closing, and/or obstructing the valve orifice. Distal thrombo-embolic phenomena may also occur. Inadequate anticoagulation or non-compliance with anticoagulation are major factors in the aetiology of this complication, which occurs at a linearized rate of 0.2–1%/patient-year. Structural failure of mechanical valves, with escape of the valve leaflet or disc, is virtually unknown with the current generation of mechanical valves. The clinical picture depends on the valve position and whether failure results in acute incompetence or obstruction. Patients are generally desperately ill with acute pulmonary oedema or cardiogenic shock. The diagnosis should be rapidly established by echocardiography. No time should be wasted in pursuing other investigations: emergency surgery may be life saving but the operative mortality rate is high.[9]

OTHER CARDIAC SURGICAL EMERGENCIES

Aortic dissection (see also Chapter 16)

Classification

Aortic dissection is classified according to the site and extent of aortic involvement. The Debakey and Stanford classifications are illustrated in figure 1. For practical purposes, Stanford type A dissections should be regarded as surgical, while Stanford type B dissections are generally managed medically.

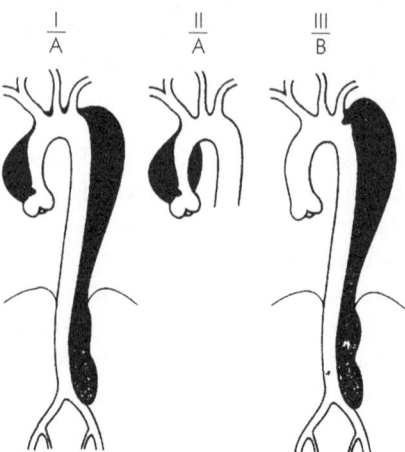

Figure 1 – Classification of aortic dissection: DeBakey types I–III and Stanford types A and B.

Clinical presentation

- Pain – severe tearing chest pain with radiation/migration to the back, abdomen or legs is typical of aortic dissection but is only present in about 50% of cases.

- Ischaemic sequelae – range from acute limb ischaemia, neurologic deficits including hemiplegia, quadriplegia or paraplegia to acute abdomen or acute renal failure, depending on the peripheral artery affected.

- Shock.

- Cardiac sequelae – myocardial infarction, from dissection of the coronaries, or acute aortic regurgitation may occur. Rupture of the dissection into the pericardium results in haemopericardium and sudden death. Rupture into the chest cavity usually results in a left-sided haemothorax, with acute circulatory collapse.

Diagnosis

- Chest X-ray – widening of the mediastinum, with or without left pleural effusion.

- Transoesophageal echocardiography (TOE) – now the investigation of choice. It has the advantages of being readily available at the patient's bedside, rapid, and highly sensitive and specific in experienced hands. Besides confirming the presence of an intraluminal flap (see Chapter 8, figure 5), TOE also provides information on left ventricular function, aortic or mitral regurgitation, and proximal main coronary arteries, all of which are important for the preoperative evaluation of patients.

- CT scan – current generation spiral CT scanners can rapidly and reliably diagnosing aortic dissection, with a sensitivity and specificity equivalent to that obtained by TOE.[10] In hospitals without ready access to TOE, CT scanning is the investigation of choice.

- MRI scan – high sensitivity and specificity for the diagnosis of aortic dissection,[11] but is not widely used due to the long scan times (30–60 min), lack of availability and requirement for only non-ferrous substances in the vicinity of an ill patient who requires intensive monitoring and constant haemodynamic care. More ideally suited for the diagnosis of equivocal cases, and for the long-term follow-up of aortic dissection.

- Aortography – the classical gold standard for the diagnosis of aortic dissection, although modern techniques have superseded this investigation. Has a sensitivity of 82–98% and a specificity about 100%, and is the procedure of choice when peripheral vascular occlusion has occurred. Contrary to common belief, retrograde aortography can be performed safely in the presence of aortic dissection, with complication rates similar to those obtained in the non-dissected aorta.

Management

Supportive therapy should be primarily aimed at pain relief and control of blood pressure as the patient is prepared for theatre and definitive investigations performed.

Type A aortic dissection is a genuine cardiac surgical emergency and definitive surgical repair should be considered in all cases. Operative mortality rate is high and ranges from 10 to 30%, mostly from exsanguination or acute cardiac failure.

Cardiac trauma

Injury to the heart should be considered in patients with both penetrating and blunt injuries to the chest, neck and upper abdomen. Although severe injuries are often rapidly fatal, with a 50–80% prehospital mortality rate,[12] a proportion of patients survive to reach hospital and can be salvaged by emergency surgery. At the other end of the spectrum, minor injuries may cause no more than transient arrhythmias or subclinical enzyme abnormalities.

Penetrating injuries of the heart

Clinical presentation

Knives, bullets or other projectiles cause the majority of civilian penetrating injuries of the heart. Iatrogenic injuries may occur in pacemaker insertion, pericardiocentesis or rarely during cardiac catheterization. Penetrating injuries may present as cardiac tamponade or exsanguination, depending on whether blood loss is contained.

Cardiac tamponade is characterized by profound shock – pallor, cool peripheries, hypotension, tachycardia, tachypnoea, restlessness, agitation, oliguria – associated with a high jugular venous pressure, disproportionately small observed blood loss and refractoriness to volume replacement or vasoconstriction. Some patients are moribund and have no detectable signs of life, while others are relatively stable and may cast doubts about whether there has been any cardiac injury. The clinical course is determined by the amount of blood in the pericardium and its rate of accumulation, which in turn is determined by the nature of the injury and its location, and whether clot formation or free bleeding into the pleural cavity occurs. If time allows, diagnostic echocardiography can be useful in establishing the presence of fluid in the pericardium, and pericardiocentesis may provide dramatic but temporary stabilization as the patient is transferred to theatre. Occasionally, associated intra-cardiac injuries, e.g.. traumatic VSD or valve injuries, may be detected.

Management

Patients with suspected penetrating injuries of the heart who present with circulatory collapse should be resuscitated aggressively and prepared for immediate surgery. Moribund patients may require emergency sternotomy or thoracotomy in the emergency room. Relief of cardiac tamponade often results in immediate haemodynamic improvement, and digital control of bleeding from the cardiac wound or direct repair prevents further decompensation. Patients with suspected penetrating injuries of the heart who present with a stable circulation should undergo diagnostic echocardiography with or without pericardiocentesis – it is important to note that pericardiocentesis may yield false-negative or positive results in up to 37% of patients with cardiac tamponade.[13] In all cases the patient should be transferred to theatre for exploration and definitive repair if there is blood in the pericardium. Patients with intra-cardiac injuries may require definitive repair under cardiopulmonary bypass.

Blunt injuries of the heart

Cardiac contusion can arise from any direct or indirect force to the chest or abdomen and most commonly arises as a result of road traffic accidents. Severe injuries are frequently associated with trauma to other organ systems, which may direct attention from the cardiac injury. It has been reported as the injury most often responsible for fatalities in these patients, with an incidence of up to 75% in severely injured patients. The spectrum of injury depends on the force of the blow and ranges from minor lacerations, petechial haemorrhage or bruising to valvular disruption, myocardial failure and fatal cardiac rupture or tamponade.[14] Epicardial coronary arteries are usually spared in blunt trauma, but rarely injuries may cause myocardial infarction or angina. Ventricular ectopics, and atrial flutter or fibrilla-tion are common, and conduction abnormalities including complete heart block may occur. In severe injuries, a common mode of death is ventricular tachycardia or fibrillation. ECG changes are non-specific, and may not appear until 24–48 h after injury. Cardiac enzymes are helpful but not diagnostic. The investigation of choice is echocardiography, which allows detailed examination for injuries to intracardiac structures and regional wall motion abnormalities. Most patients with blunt injuries to the heart can be managed by monitoring and supportive therapy; only the rare patient with intracardiac lesions requires urgent or emergency surgery.

Traumatic aortic rupture

One of the commonest reasons for referrals to the cardiothoracic service after road traffic accidents is the 'broadened mediastinum'. It brings with it fears of traumatic aortic injury and visions of sudden death by exsanguination. The frequency of this injury has increased in recent decades due to the increase in incidence of high-speed road traffic accidents. Probably 15–20% of mortally injured road traffic acci-dent victims will have traumatic aortic rupture. Associated injuries are common: an incidence of 2.9 major fractures, 3.9 major organ injuries[15] and 48% major intra-abdominal injury requiring laparotomy[16] have been reported.

The injury may occur after severe deceleration of any description, either horizon-tal as in a road traffic accident, or vertical as after free fall. Extreme compressive or crush injuries to the chest may also result in aortic rupture. Four separate mecha-nisms have been proposed to account for the injury and its two characteristic sites: at the aortic isthmus (50–60%), shearing stress from differential deceleration of the relatively fixed descending aorta as opposed to the mobile aortic arch and heart, or bending stress at the left main bronchus and left pulmonary artery. In the ascend-ing aorta (10–20%), torsional stress created by sudden displacement of the heart into the left chest, and the water hammer effect created by an abrupt rise in intra-aortic pressure may result in traumatic rupture. Of patients who survive to undergo surgery, 95% have isolated aortic rupture at the isthmus. As might be expected from the nature of the injury, traumatic aortic rupture is a highly lethal injury that is 80–85% fatal at the time of the accident. If the patient survives > 30 min, 21% will die in the next 6 h, 32% will die in the next 24 h, 60% will die within 1 week, and 90% will die within 10 weeks.

Clinical presentation

The symptoms of traumatic aortic rupture are non-specific and include chest pain, mid-scapular pain, dyspnoea, and rarely hoarseness, dysphagia and ischaemic sequelae to upper limbs, head or spinal cord. Commonly the symptoms and signs of associated injuries dominate the clinical picture, especially as > 50% of patients present with no external evidence of severe chest trauma. Three physical signs are of importance: upper limb hypertension, pulse amplitude difference between upper and lower extremities ('pseudocoarctation'), and a systolic murmur over the precordium or the mid-scapular area attributed to turbulent blood flow in the region of the rupture.

Diagnosis

CXR – abnormal in > 90% of patients, although a normal CXR does not exclude aortic rupture:

- Widening of superior mediastinum.

- Loss of sharpness of aortic outline.

- Obscurity of aortic knob.

- Obliteration of the aortopulmonary window.

- Obscuration of medial aspect of left upper lobe.

- Depression of left main bronchus.

- Displacement of trachea or oesophagus to right.

- Left pleural effusion/haemothorax.

- Widening of paravertebral stripe.

Associated injuries:

- First or second rib fracture.

- Fractured sternum.

- Fracture or dislocation of thoracic spine.

Unfortunately there is no good definition and considerable observer variability in the reporting of mediastinal widening.[17] Patients presenting with the above clinical and radiological findings who have a compatible history of a high-speed deceleration injury must therefore undergo further diagnostic investigations.

Contrast CT

This is a good screening investigation that is often diagnostic and has the advantage of also being useful in the examination of other injuries in the multiply injured patient. However, reported sensitivity ranges from 55 to 100% and specificity from 40 to 96%. While a negative scan is reliable in haemodynamically stable patients with a normal CXR, contrast CT should be regarded in most as a screening investigation to determine the need to proceed to angiography.[18]

Transoesophageal echocardiography

In experienced hands transoesophageal echocardiography has a sensitivity of 100% and a specificity of 99–100%. However, the technique has not gained wide acceptance in patients with multiple trauma due to the risk of aspiration, or technical difficulties in those with facial or cervical spinal fractures.

Aortography

This remains the gold standard for the diagnosis of traumatic aortic rupture, and should be undertaken in all cases where the diagnosis still remains in doubt despite the above investigations. Typically, traumatic aortic transection appears as a pseudo-aneurysm near the isthmus, although complete aortic interruption may occur. This investigation, if performed through the femoral approach, carries the theoretical risk of iatrogenic dissection or rupture of the aorta from passage of the angiographic catheter.

Treatment

Surgical repair should be undertaken in almost all cases, unless concomitant injuries render the patient unsalvageable. These injuries, if life-threatening, should be treated first. The prioritization of treatment and the formulation of a successful management strategy depend on a multidisciplinary team effort, and a common sense approach to the multiply injured patient. Despite advances in surgical techniques and intensive care in recent years, the mortality rate of this condition remains high, ranging from 25 to 50% in reported series.

Massive pulmonary embolus

Clinical presentation

Massive pulmonary embolism is one of the most feared complications of childbirth and major surgery, and may present as sudden death or circulatory failure. Syncope or collapse occurs in 80%; acute respiratory failure in 70%; and central chest pain in 35% of patients. Physical signs are non-specific and include tachypnoea, tachycardia, cyanosis, hypotension, a prominent 'a' wave in the JVP, a powerful parasternal lift, a right heart gallop and accentuation of the pulmonary second sound. The legs should always be examined for the signs of deep vein thrombosis (DVT), although it should be recognized that 70% of DVT give rise to neither symptom nor signs.

Diagnosis

Massive pulmonary embolism mimics a variety of other medical emergencies and its diagnosis depends on a high index of suspicion in susceptible patients.

- Chest X-ray – may be normal. There may be oligaemia of the affected lung or an abnormally enlarged pulmonary artery. Occasionally, the pulmonary artery may be seen to terminate abruptly.

- ECG:

  S1 Q3 T3

  new right bundle branch block

  myocardial ischaemia may result from coronary hypoperfusion

  non-specific sinus tachycardia, supraventricular tachycardia or atrial fibrillation

- Arterial blood gases confirm respiratory failure with a $PO_2 = \; < 8.0$ kPa, hypocapnoea and acidosis.

- Contrast CT scan.

- Pulmonary angiography.

Management

Supportive therapy includes oxygen by facemask and IV fluids to maintain a high right-sided ventricular filling pressure. Desperately ill patients require intubation and ventilation. Inotropic agents may be required to support the failing right heart. Definitive therapy may be medical by thrombolysis or surgical by emergency pulmonary embolectomy. Cardiopulmonary bypass is preferable but not essential. Most patients with pulmonary embolism can, and should be, managed medically. Surgical treatment should be considered in patients who are haemodynamically compromised, in those in whom thrombolytic therapy is contraindicated, and in those in whom the inherent delays in attempted thrombolysis is judged unacceptable.[19] Operative mortality rate is high, especially in patients who been resuscitated from an episode of cardiac asystole or ventricular fibrillation (60–70%); those who do not present with cardiac arrest have an operative mortality rate of 20%.[20]

Mechanical cardiac assist

Over the past 30 years, a variety of circulatory support devices have been developed for the temporary support of patients with terminal heart failure. These devices range from the intra-aortic balloon pump (see Chapter 9), designed for short-term assist of the failing heart, but unable in itself totally to supplant ventricular function, to total artificial hearts designed to substitute the biological heart. In between are various ventricular assist devices that can supplant completely the function of the left or right ventricle, and which may be extracorporeal or completely implantable. With advances in technology and improvements in performance, the indications for the implantation of such devices have evolved. Currently, ventricular assist devices are implanted acutely in post-cardiotomy myocardial failure as a bridge to recovery, or urgently in end-stage cardiac failure as a bridge to recovery (e.g.. in acute viral myocarditis), a bridge to transplantation, or as a long-term alternative to transplantation. Clinical results are encouraging: about 30–40% of patients are successfully bridged to recovery, and 60–70% successfully bridged to transplantation. Patients with long-term implantable ventricular assist devices have a reasonable quality of life, on a par with renal transplant recipients.[21] Up to 2 years of complete ventricular support has been reported. The running costs of these devices are very high, and in the impoverished NHS is only affordable in very few centres in the UK as part of ongoing research.

References

1. UK Cardiac Surgery Registry: Minimum Surgical Dataset Definitions [URL: www.scts.org].

2. Patel D. Current diagnostic and therapeutic strategies in unstable angina. *Br J Cardiol* 1999; **6**: 680–91.

3. Brown CA, Hutter AM, De Sanctis RW *et al.* Prospective study of medical and urgent surgical therapy in randomisable patients with unstable angina pectoris: results of in-hospital and chronic mortality and morbidity. *Am Heart J* 1981; **102**: 959–64.

4. Agency for Health Care Policy and Research, National Heart, Lung and Blood Institute. *Unstable Angina: Diagnosis and Management.* Clinical Practice Guideline no. 10., AHCPR publication no. 94–0602. Rockville: US Department of Health and Human Services, Public Health Service, 1994.

5. Westaby S, Parry A, Ormerod O *et al.* Thrombolysis and postinfarction ventricular septal rupture. *J Thorac Cardiovasc Surg* 1992; **104**: 1506–9.

6. Jones MT, Schofield PM, Dark JF *et al.* Surgical repair of acquired ventricular septal defect. Determinants of early and late outcome. *J Thorac Cardiovac Surg* 1987; **93**: 680–6.

7. Kirklin JW, Barratt-Boyes BG. Left ventricular aneurysm. In *Cardiac Surgery*, 2nd edn. New York: Churchill Livingstone, 1993: 383–402.

8. Schoen FJ. Modes of failure and other pathology of mechanical and tissue heart valve prostheses. In Bodnar E, Frater R (eds), *Replacement Cardiac Valves.* New York: McGraw-Hill, 1992: 99–124.

9. Au J, Sang CTM. Strut fracture and disc embolisation of a Bjork–Shiley aortic prosthesis: emergency operation with survival. *Scan J Thorac Cardiovasc Surg* 1989; **23**: 297–8.

10. Nienaber CA, von Kodolitsch Y, Nicolas V *et al*. The diagnosis of thoracic aortic dissection by non-invasive imaging procedures. *N Engl J Med* 1993; **328**: 1–9.

11. Panting JR, Norell MS, Baker C, Nicholson AR. Feasibility, accuracy and safety of magnetic resonance imaging in acute aortic dissection. *Clin Radiol* 1995; **50**: 455–8.

12. Culliford AT. Penetrating cardiac injuries. In Hood RM, Boyd AD, Culliford AT (eds), *Thoracic Trauma*. Philadelphia: WB Saunders, 1989: 178–210.

13. DeGennaro VA, Bonfils-Roberts EA, Ching N, Nealon TF Jr. Aggressive management of potential penetrating cardiac injuries. *J Thorac Cardiovasc Surg* 1980; **79**: 833–7.

14. Culliford AT. Nonpenetrating cardiac trauma. In Hood RM, Boyd AD, Culliford AT (eds), *Thoracic Trauma*. Philadelphia: WB Saunders, 1989: 211–23

15. Greendyke RM. Traumatic rupture of the aorta: special reference to automobile accidents. *J Am Med Assoc* 1966; **195**: 527–30.

16. Borman KR, Aurbakken CM, Weigelt JA. Treatment priorities in combined blunt abdominal and aortic trauma. *Am J Surg* 1982; **144**: 728–32.

17. Gundry SR, Burney RE, MacKenzie JR *et al*. Assessment of mediastinal widening associated with traumatic rupture of the aorta. *J Trauma* 1983; **23**: 293–9.

18. Driscoll PA, Hyde JAJ, Curzon I *et al*. Traumatic disruption of the thoracic aorta: a rational approach to imaging. *Injury* 1996; **27**: 679–85.

19. Beall AC. Pulmonary embolectomy. *Ann Thorac Surg* 1991; **51**: 179.

20. Gray HH, Miller GH, Paneth M. Pulmonary embolectomy: its place in the management of pulmonary embolism. *Lancet* 1988; **i**: 1441–5.

21. Clarke DB, Abrams LD. Pulmonary embolectomy: a 25-year experience. *J Thorac Cardiovasc Surg* 1986; **92**: 442–5.

22. Moskowitz AJ, Weinberg AD, Mehmet CO, Williams DL. Quality of life with an implanted left ventricular assist device. *Ann Thorac Surg* 1997; **64**: 1764–9.

INDEX